Workbook for

Know the Body: Muscle, Bone, and Palpation Essentials

T0195222

Joseph E. Muscolino, DC
Instructor, Purchase College
State University of New York
Purchase, New York

Owner, The Art and Science of Kinesiology
Stamford, Connecticut

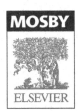
MOSBY
ELSEVIER

ELSEVIER
MOSBY

3251 Riverport Lane
St. Louis, Missouri 63043

WORKBOOK FOR KNOW THE BODY:
MUSCLE, BONE, AND PALPATION ESSENTIALS   ISBN: 978-0-323-08683-7

ISBN: 978-0-323-08683-7

Vice President and Publisher: Linda Duncan
Executive Content Strategist: Kellie White
Senior Content Development Specialist: Jennifer Watrous
Content Coordinator: Emily Thomson
Publishing Services Manager: Julie Eddy
Senior Project Manager: Andrea Campbell
Design Direction: Teresa McBryan

Printed in the United States of America

Last digit is the print number: 9 8 7 6 5 4 3

Preface

Corresponding to the chapters in Muscolino's *Know the Body: Muscle, Bone, and Palpation Essentials,* this workbook includes review activities to help students learn and apply muscle, bone, and palpation knowledge as well as features that facilitate learning. These features include the following:

1. CHAPTER-BY-CHAPTER, COMPREHENSIVE REVIEW covers all of the content from the Know the Body textbook to ensure that students are prepared for exams and for practice.

2. PHOTOS OF JOINT MOVEMENTS provide a better understanding of movement and range of motion, as compared to simple drawings.

3. A WIDE RANGE OF FUN, INTERESTING REVIEW ACTIVITIES includes structure identification and labeling, coloring, matching, true/false, multiple choice, short answer, crossword puzzle, and mnemonic fill-in-the-blanks.

4. HIGH-LEVEL EXERCISES help in developing critical thinking abilities and understanding how to apply muscle, bone, and palpation knowledge in the treatment room.

5. DOWNLOADABLE AUDIO PRONUNCIATIONS OF MUSCLES AND INTERACTIVE REVIEW EXERCISES on the Evolve companion website allow students to study anytime, anywhere.

6. PERFORATED PAGES make it easy to remove exercises from the workbook and hand in for grading.

7. ANSWERS are included at the end of the workbook, allowing students and instructors to pinpoint strengths and identify areas that need further study.

These features should make mastery of the material contained in this text and workbook a rewarding experience for both instructor and student.

How to Use the Exercises in This Workbook

After you have read a chapter and learned all the new vocabulary it contains, begin working with the workbook. Read the overview of the chapter, which summarizes the main points.

Complete the questions and diagrams in the workbook. A variety of questions is offered throughout the workbook to help you cover the material effectively. Aside from the normal multiple choice, true or false, matching, and fill-in-the-blank exercises, this workbook has several exercises you may not be familiar with. The following examples are among the exercises that have been included to assist you.

Coloring & Labeling Exercises

At the beginning of the chapters, there are Coloring & Labeling exercises that present images with structures that are not identified. For each of these images, you are to look at the numbered list of terms, choose the term that corresponds to a blank line by an unidentified structure and print the number corresponding to each structure on the line. You may choose to further distinguish the structures by coloring them with a variety of colors. After you have written down the names of all the structures to be identified, check your answers. When it comes time to review before an examination, you can place a sheet of paper over the answers you have already written on the lines. This procedure will allow you to test yourself a second time without seeing the answers.

Know Your Muscles

Each section of chapters 6-11 has an exercise that shows small pictures of different muscles. You will fill in the blank below each picture with the name of the muscle.

What's in a Name?

In this matching exercise, you will match the muscle name from the right column to its meaning in the left column. Write your answer in the space provided.

Matching Attachments

Attachments are listed in a two-column table on the left column. You will match each muscle from the word bank with its attachments. Write the answer in the column labeled Muscle. Each choice will be used only once.

The Big Picture – Functional Groups

As a rule, these questions have three blanks to fill in: 1) the direction of movement, 2) the body part that is moving, and 3) the joint at which movement occurs.

Matching Actions

Each muscle has a certain number of blanks next to it. Place the corresponding joint action letter(s) in the blank(s) next to the muscle. Some letters will be used more than once.

The Long and the Short of It Exercises

This is a two-part exercise where you will indicate muscle shortening and lengthening. In the first part, for each joint action given, indicate whether the muscle shortens or lengthens. In the second part, for each joint action given, fill in the blanks with a muscle that shortens and a muscle that lengthens.

Movers & Antagonists Exercises

This two-part exercise tests your knowledge of movers and antagonists. In the first part, for each joint action stated, fill in the blanks for a mover and antagonist of that joint action. Please choose your mover/antagonist pairs from the word bank. Each pair can be used once and only once. In the second part, for each joint action illustrated in which the body part is being *slowly* moved, circle whether the functional muscle group of the pair provided is contracting or relaxed. Then circle how the muscle group that is working is contracting (concentrically or eccentrically.)

Muscle Stabilizations

This multiple choice exercise tests your knowledge of the stabilization function of muscles.

You've got Nerve!

Write the name of the corresponding innervation from the list provided. Choices can be used more than once.

Are you Feeling It?—Palpation

These fill-in-the-blank questions test your palpation knowledge.

Clinically Speaking

These questions review the *Treatment Considerations* sections of the *Know the Body* textbook.

Muscle Mash-Up

Muscle Mash-Up is a review of all aspects of muscle knowledge.

Crossword Puzzles

Vocabulary words from the chapter of the text have been developed into crossword puzzles. This format encourages both recall and proper spelling.

Mini Case Studies

Brief case studies are presented to test your ability to apply muscle knowledge to clinical scenarios.

Reviewing Your Answers

After completing the exercises in the workbook, check your answers. If they are not correct, refer to the text chapter and review it for further clarification. If you still do not understand the question or the answer, ask your instructor for further explanation.

ACKNOWLEDGMENTS

The longer I have written, the more I have come to realize what a collaborative effort a book is. I am so very lucky to have a great team behind me at Elsevier. This is my chance to thank all these wonderful people. To begin with, this book is a workbook that accompanies *Know the Body: Muscle, Bone, and Palpation Essentials*. Therefore, I must begin by thanking everyone who assisted me in the creation of that book.

Specifically, I have a wonderful art team: Jean Luciano of Connecticut, Jeanne Robertson of Missouri, Frank Forney and David Carlson of Colorado, Peter Bull of England, and Jodie Bernard and Giovanni Rimasti of Lightbox Visuals out of our wonderful neighbor to the North, Canada. Superb photography was done by Yanik Chauvin, also out of Canada.

My team at Elsevier was, as usual, amazing and wonderful to work with. At this point in time, they feel like family. Kellie White, my acquisitions editor; Jennifer Watrous and Emily Thomson, my developmental editors; and Andrea Campbell, my production editor. I must also thank Chris Jones, Selena Anduze, Celia Bucci, Neal Delaporta, and Kenneth Hewes for helping me to organize much of the content in this workbook.

A continual thank you to William Courtland, a previous student and now fellow instructor, who one day, many years ago said: "You should write a book." Those words launched my writing career.

And, as always, my tremendous love and appreciation to everyone in my family, especially Simona Cipriani, my angel, my love, and my partner in life.

Table of Contents

1 | Basic Kinesiology Terminology

MAJOR BODY PARTS

COLORING & LABELING

Use crayons or felt-tipped markers to color the parts of the body. Use the word bank to fill in the numbers that correspond to the names of the parts of the body in the blanks provided.

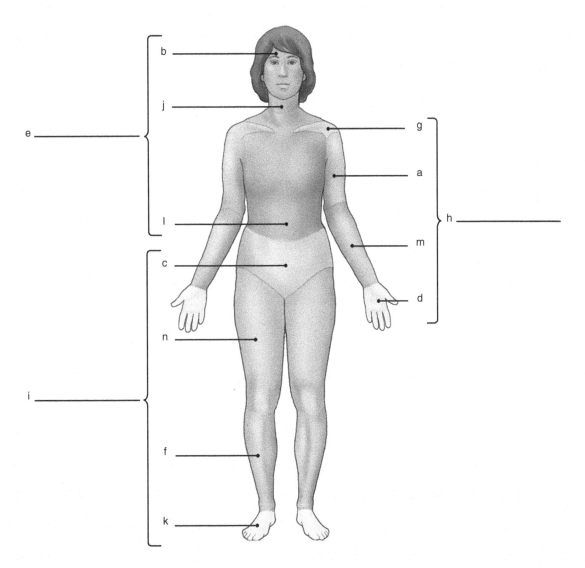

1. Arm
2. Axial body parts
3. Foot
4. Forearm
5. Hand
6. Head
7. Leg
8. Lower extremity body parts
9. Neck
10. Pelvis
11. Shoulder girdle
12. Thigh
13. Trunk
14. Upper extremity body parts

Score: ___/14

1

MATCHING

Match the anatomic description on the left with the proper body part on the right. Write your answer in the space provided. Each choice will be used only once.

Anatomic Description

_____ 1. Shoulder joint to elbow joint

_____ 2. Elbow joint to wrist joint

_____ 3. Distal to wrist joint

_____ 4. Between trunk and thighs

_____ 5. Hip joint to knee joint

_____ 6. Knee joint to ankle joint

_____ 7. Distal to ankle joint

Body Part

a. Thigh

b. Pelvis

c. Foot

d. Leg

e. Forearm

f. Arm

g. Hand

Score: ___/7

TRUE OR FALSE

Write T on the line if the statement is true or F if the statement is false.

1. _____ The thigh is part of the leg.

2. _____ The forearm is part of the arm.

3. _____ The pelvis is part of the trunk.

4. _____ The appendicular body is composed of the upper and lower extremities.

5. _____ The hand is distal to the forearm.

6. _____ The neck is superior to the trunk.

7. _____ The foot is proximal to the leg.

Score: ___/7

FILL IN THE BLANK

Fill in the blank with the answer that best completes each question or statement.

1. The _____ and _____ are the two major subdivisions of the body.

2. Between which two joints is the leg located?_____ & _____.

3. The _____ body part is immediately inferior to the trunk.

4. The _____ body part is immediately proximal to the hand.

5. The _____ body part is immediately distal to the thigh.

Score: ___/5

MULTIPLE CHOICE

Circle the letter of the best answer to the question.

1. Where is the pelvis located?
   a. Directly between the trunk and thighs
   b. Directly between the trunk and legs
   c. It is the inferior aspect of the trunk
   d. Distal to the legs

2. How is the location of the leg best described?
   a. Inferior to the thigh
   b. Superior to the foot
   c. Lateral to the other leg
   d. Distal to the thigh

3. What are the two major subdivisions of the body?
   a. Legs and arms
   b. Trunk and axial
   c. Axial and appendicular
   d. Right and left

4. What are the parts of an upper extremity?
   a. Upper arm, lower arm, hand
   b. Shoulder girdle, arm, hand
   c. Shoulder girdle, arm, forearm, hand
   d. Arm, forearm, hand

5. What are the parts of a lower extremity?
   a. Leg, foot
   b. Pelvis, thigh, leg, foot
   c. Thigh, leg, foot
   d. Upper leg, lower leg, foot

Score: ___/5

Use the clues to complete the crossword puzzle.

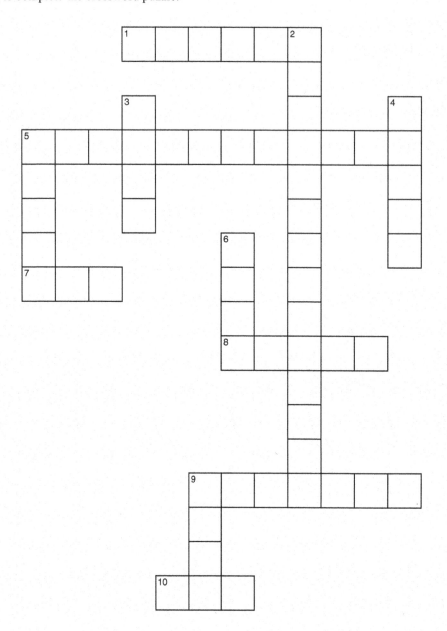

ACROSS

1 Proximal to the thigh
5 Upper and lower extremities
7 Distal to the thigh
8 Between hip joint and knee joint
9 Proximal to the hand
10 Between shoulder joint and elbow joint

DOWN

2 Scapula and clavicle (2 words)
3 Superior to the neck
4 Between neck and pelvis
5 Appendicular and _____
6 Most distal part of lower extremity
9 Number of major parts in an upper extremity

Score: ___/12

NAME THE POINT

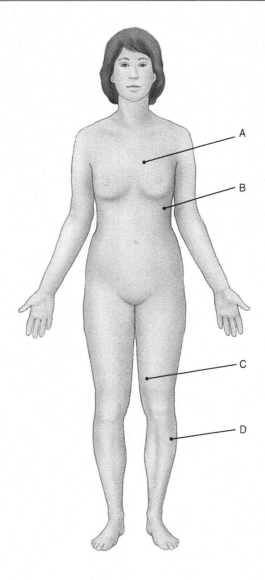

1. WHERE IS POINT A IN RELATION TO POINT B? _____ & _____

2. WHERE IS POINT D IN RELATION TO POINT C? _____ & _____

Score: ___/2

MATCHING

Match the corresponding pairs of terms. Write your answer in the space provided. Some choices may be used more than once.

_____ 1. Anterior

_____ 2. Medial

_____ 3. Superior

_____ 4. Proximal

_____ 5. Ventral

_____ 6. Superficial

_____ 7. Radial

_____ 8. Tibial

_____ 9. Palmar

_____ 10. Plantar

_____ 11. Cranial

a. Dorsal (used three times)

b. Caudal

c. Posterior

d. Deep

e. Inferior

f. Lateral

g. Fibular

h. Distal

i. Ulnar

Score: ___/11

TRUE OR FALSE

Write T on the line if the statement is true or F if the statement is false.

1. _____ The knee is inferior to the thigh.

2. _____ All movements begin from the anatomic position.

3. _____ The belly button is inferior to the sternum.

4. _____ The little finger is lateral to the thumb.

5. _____ The wrist is distal to the arm.

6. _____ The nipple is superolateral to the belly button.

7. _____ The nose is inferolateral to the eye.

Score: ___/7

FILL IN THE BLANK

Fill in the blank with the answer that best completes each question or statement.

1. The _____ is the reference position for location terminology (naming structures on the body and points on the body).

2. Where on the body can the terms anterior and posterior be used? _____

6

3. The terms plantar and dorsal are used in reference to the _____.

4. The term _____ is sometimes used instead or in place of anterior.

5. The term _____ is usually used in place of superior on the appendicular body.

MULTIPLE CHOICE

Circle the letter of the best answer to the question.

1. Which of the following describes anatomic position? The person is standing erect with…
   a. Arms at the sides, palms facing posteriorly, fingers and toes extended
   b. Arms abducted, palms facing anteriorly, fingers extended, toes flexed
   c. Arms at the sides, palms facing anteriorly, fingers and toes extended
   d. Arms abducted, palms facing posteriorly, fingers and toes flexed

2. On which side of the hand is the thumb located?
   a. Radial/lateral
   b. Radial/medial
   c. Ulnar/lateral
   d. Ulnar/medial

3. What term describes a location closer to the front of the body?
   a. Lateral
   b. Medial
   c. Superior
   d. Anterior

4. What term describes a location closer to the midline of the body?
   a. Medial
   b. Lateral
   c. Radial
   d. Caudal

5. Points A and B are on the axial body. If point A is closer to the front, farther from the midline, and higher than point B, then how do we describe the location of point A relative to point B?
   a. Posteromedial and inferior
   b. Anterolateral and superior
   c. Anteromedial and superior
   d. Anterolateral and inferior

Use the clues to complete the crossword puzzle.

ACROSS

2 Radius relative to ulna
3 Location of heart relative
   to sternum
5 Bottom of foot
6 Closer to the surface of the body
10 Closer to the midline of the body
11 More lateral bone of leg
12 In anatomic position, the hands
   face_____

DOWN

1 Higher on the leg
4 Toward the back of the body
7 Front of the hand
8 Superior versus _____
9 Closer to the front

Score: ___/12

Chapter **1 Basic Kinesiology Terminology**   Copyright © 2013 by Mosby, an imprint of Elsevier Inc. All rights reserved.

NAME THE PLANE OR AXIS

Name the plane in each figure.

1.

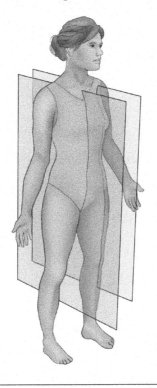
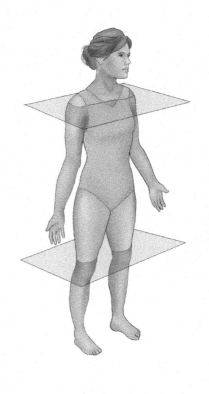

_____   _____

Identify the corresponding axis for the plane shown in each figure.

2.

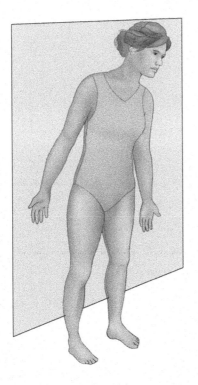
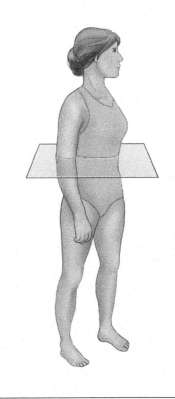

_____   _____

Score: ___/2

9

Chapter **1** **Basic Kinesiology Terminology**

MATCHING

Match the movement term pairs with the corresponding plane (Column A) in which the movement occurs from and the corresponding axis (Column B) around which motion occurs from. Choices from each column can be used more than once.

Column A: Plane

Sagittal

Oblique

Transverse

Frontal

Column B: Axis

Oblique

Mediolateral

Anteroposterior

Superoinferior

Description of Movement	Name of plane	Corresponding axis
Vertical: anterior to posterior	_____	_____
Vertical: side to side	_____	_____
Horizontal	_____	_____
Oblique	_____	_____

Score: ___/4

TRUE OR FALSE

Write T on the line if the statement is true or F if the statement is false.

1. _____ All three cardinal planes are vertical.

2. _____ The orientation of an axis to its corresponding plane is always perpendicular.

3. _____ The axis for the sagittal plane is anteroposterior.

4. _____ Axial motion of a body part is circular.

5. _____ Motion within the transverse plane is horizontal.

Score: ___/5

FILL IN THE BLANK

Fill in the blank with the answer that best completes each question or statement.

1. The _____, _____, and _____ are the three cardinal planes.

2. A(n) _____ is an imaginary line around which a body part moves.

3. What is the importance of planes? _____

4. What are the three cardinal axes? _____

5. The term _____ describes motion that occurs within a plane and around an axis.

Score: ___/5

Chapter 1 **Basic Kinesiology Terminology**

MULTIPLE CHOICE

Circle the letter of the best answer to the question.

1. What is the corresponding axis for the frontal plane?
   a. Vertical
   b. Superoinferior
   c. Mediolateral
   d. Anteroposterior

2. What is the corresponding axis for the transverse plane?
   a. Oblique
   b. Vertical
   c. Anteroposterior
   d. Mediolateral

3. What is another name for the vertical axis?
   a. Superoinferior
   b. Mediolateral
   c. Anteroposterior
   d. None of the above

4. Which of the following is true regarding an oblique plane?
   a. It has components of two or three cardinal planes.
   b. Its axis is vertical.
   c. It divides the body into superior and inferior halves.
   d. All of the above

5. What kind of motion occurs within the sagittal plane?
   a. Vertical
   b. Horizontal
   c. Oblique
   d. None of the above

Score: ___/5

Use the clues to complete the crossword puzzle.

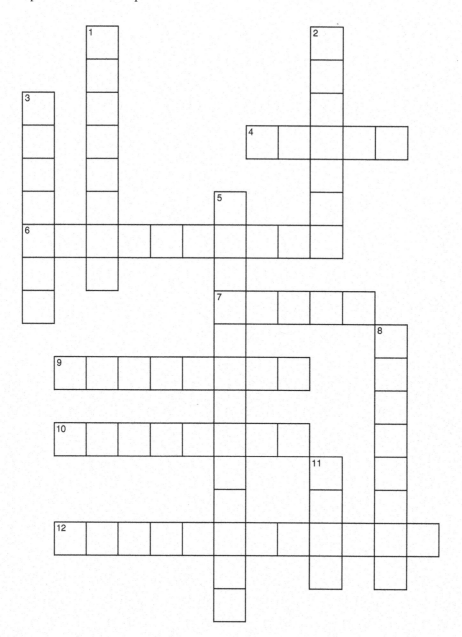

ACROSS

4 Circular motion
6 Divides the body into superior
   and inferior portions
7 Maps 3D space
9 Major planes
10 Straight line motion
12 Sagittal plane axis

DOWN

1 Transverse plane axis
2 Plane that is not perfectly cardinal
3 Divides the body into front and back
   portions
5 Orientation of cardinal plane to other
   cardinal planes
8 Divides the body into left and right
   portions
11 Plural of axis

Score: ___/12

NAME THE MOTION

Identify the movements occurring on the lines below the figures.

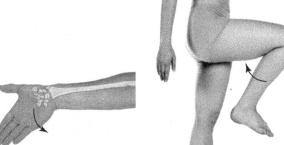

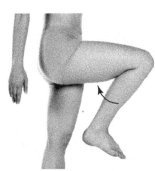

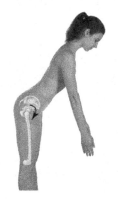

a: _____

of the _____

at the _____ joint(s)

b: _____

of the _____

at the _____ joint(s)

c: _____

of the _____

at the _____ joint(s)

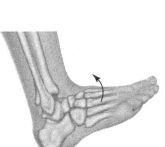

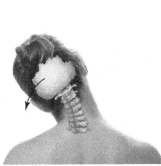

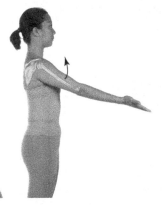

d: _____

of the _____

at the _____ joint(s)

e: _____

of the _____

at the _____ joint(s)

f: _____

of the _____

at the _____ joint(s)

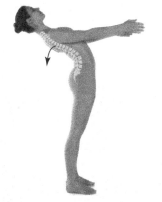

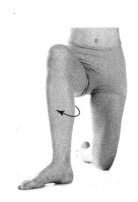

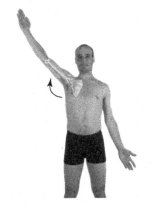

g: _____

of the _____

at the _____ joint(s)

h: _____

of the _____

at the _____ joint(s)

i: _____

of the _____

at the _____ joint(s)

Score: ___/9

13

MATCHING

Match the movement term pairs with the corresponding plane (Column A) in which the movement occurs and the corresponding axis (Column B) around which the movement occurs. Choices from each column can be used more than once.

Column A: Plane

Frontal

Transverse

Sagittal

Column B: Axis

Vertical

Mediolateral

Anteroposterior

Movement	**Plane**	**Axis**
Flexion/Extension	_____	_____
Abduction/Adduction	_____	_____
Right lateral flexion/Left lateral flexion	_____	_____
Left rotation/Right rotation	_____	_____
Lateral rotation	_____	_____
Dorsiflexion/Plantarflexion	_____	_____

Score: ___/6

TRUE OR FALSE

Write T on the line if the statement is true or F if the statement is false.

1. _____ Circumduction is an action.

2. _____ Horizontal flexion is also known as horizontal adduction.

3. _____ Upward and downward rotations of the scapula must occur with actions of the arm at the glenohumeral joint.

4. _____ Opposition of the thumb is one cardinal plane action.

5. _____ Dorsiflexion of the foot at the ankle joint is flexion.

Score: ___/5

FILL IN THE BLANK

Fill in the blank with the answer that best completes each question or statement.

1. The term _____ describes extension that is beyond the healthy or normal extension range of motion.

2. Which two body parts can pronate? _____ & _____

3. If a muscle on the right side of the body can rotate a body part to the left side of the body, then that muscle can be described as a(n) _____.

4. What do joint actions usually describe? _____

5. _____ occurs when the pad of the thumb meets the pad of another finger.

MULTIPLE CHOICE

Circle the letter of the best answer to the question.

1. At which joint does the foot invert?
   a. Ankle
   b. Subtalar
   c. Both A and B
   d. None of the above

2. Which of the following pairs of terms is used only in the axial body?
   a. Abduction/Adduction
   b. Right rotation/Left rotation
   c. Lateral rotation/Medial rotation
   d. Flexion/Extension

3. Which of the following pairs of terms is used only in the appendicular body?
   a. Flexion/Extension
   b. Right lateral flexion/Left lateral flexion
   c. Right rotation/Left rotation
   d. Abduction/Adduction

4. Which of the following statements is true regarding pronation of the foot?
   a. Pronation is eversion.
   b. Pronation is inversion.
   c. The principal component of pronation is eversion.
   d. The principal component of pronation is inversion.

5. What does the term *hyper* mean?
   a. Too little
   b. Normal amount
   c. Too much
   d. None of the above

Chapter **1** **Basic Kinesiology Terminology**

Use the clues to complete the crossword puzzle.

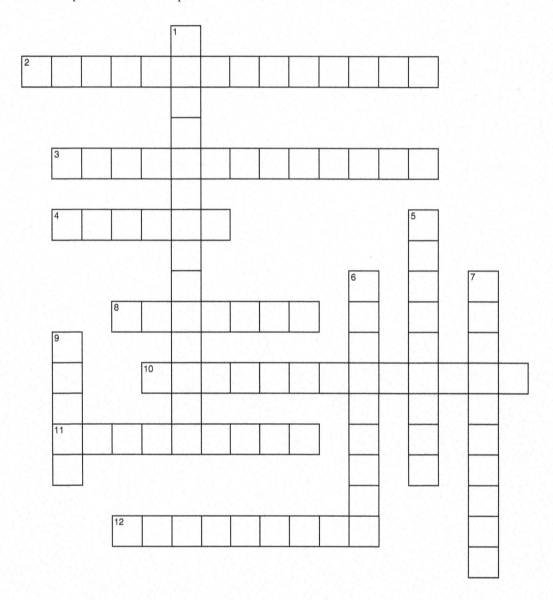

ACROSS

2 Anterior surface comes to face the midline (2 words)
3 Anterior surface comes to face to the right (2 words)
4 Rotation that faces the glenoid fossa more superiorly
8 Usually moves a body part more anteriorly
10 Sequence of four actions
11 Usually moves a body part more posteriorly
12 Toward midline

DOWN

1 Flexion of foot
5 Upward motion
6 Away from midline
7 Saddle joint motion
9 Too much

Score: ___/12

COLORING & LABELING

Use crayons or felt-tipped markers to color the bones. Use the word banks to fill in the numbers that correspond to the names of the bones and bony landmarks in the blanks provided.

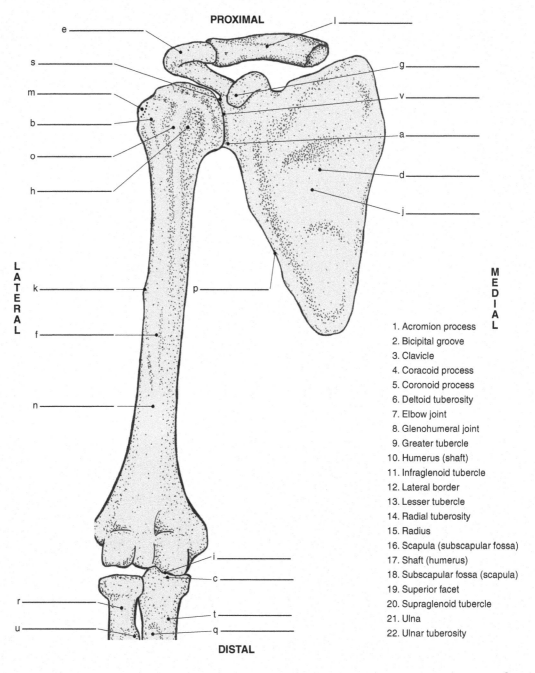

1. Acromion process
2. Bicipital groove
3. Clavicle
4. Coracoid process
5. Coronoid process
6. Deltoid tuberosity
7. Elbow joint
8. Glenohumeral joint
9. Greater tubercle
10. Humerus (shaft)
11. Infraglenoid tubercle
12. Lateral border
13. Lesser tubercle
14. Radial tuberosity
15. Radius
16. Scapula (subscapular fossa)
17. Shaft (humerus)
18. Subscapular fossa (scapula)
19. Superior facet
20. Supraglenoid tubercle
21. Ulna
22. Ulnar tuberosity

Score: ___/22

17

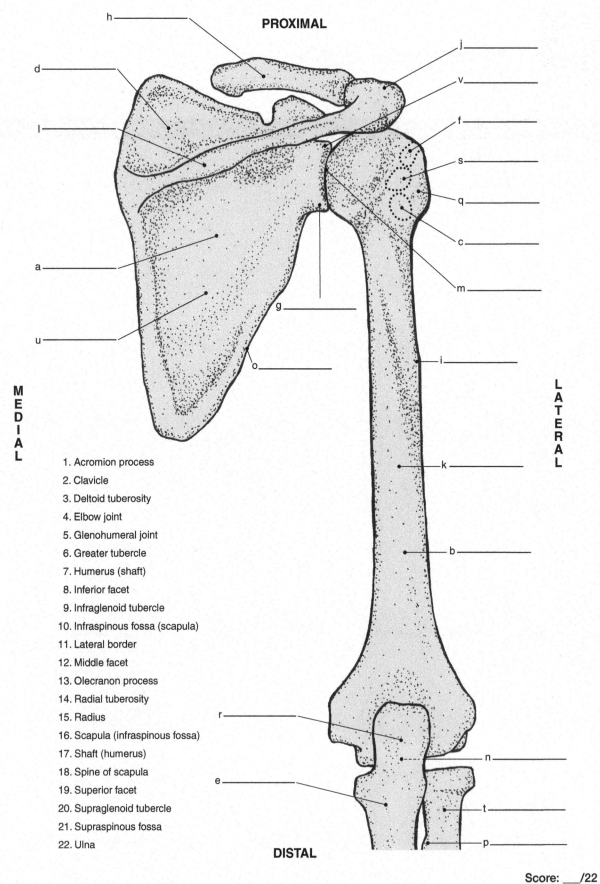

PROXIMAL

h

d

l

a

u

MEDIAL

j

v

f

s

q

c

m

LATERAL

g

o

i

k

b

r

e

n

t

p

DISTAL

1. Acromion process
2. Clavicle
3. Deltoid tuberosity
4. Elbow joint
5. Glenohumeral joint
6. Greater tubercle
7. Humerus (shaft)
8. Inferior facet
9. Infraglenoid tubercle
10. Infraspinous fossa (scapula)
11. Lateral border
12. Middle facet
13. Olecranon process
14. Radial tuberosity
15. Radius
16. Scapula (infraspinous fossa)
17. Shaft (humerus)
18. Spine of scapula
19. Superior facet
20. Supraglenoid tubercle
21. Supraspinous fossa
22. Ulna

Score: ___/22

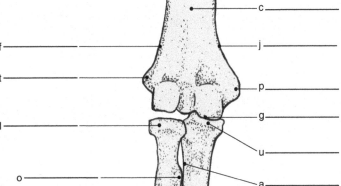

PROXIMAL

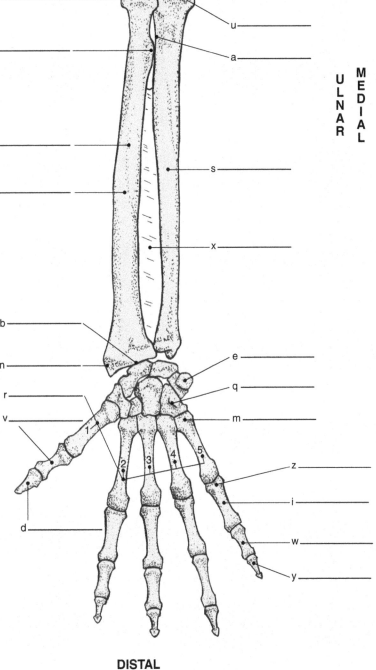

LATERAL **RADIAL**

ULNAR **MEDIAL**

c

f

j

t

p

l

g

u

o

a

h

s

k

x

b

n

e

q

r

m

v

z

i

d

w

y

1. Base of metacarpal
2. Base of phalanx
3. Coronoid process
4. Distal phalanx of finger
5. Distal phalanx of thumb
6. Elbow joint
7. Head of radius
8. Hook of hamate
9. Humerus
10. Interosseus membrane
11. Lateral epicondyle
12. Lateral supracondylar ridge
13. Medial epicondyle
14. Medial supracondylar ridge
15. Metacarpals
16. Middle phalanx of finger
17. Pisiform
18. Proximal phalanx of finger
19. Proximal phalanx of thumb
20. Radial shaft (radius)
21. Radial tuberosity
22. Radius (radial shaft)
23. Styloid process of radius
24. Supinator crest
25. Ulna
26. Wrist joint

DISTAL

Score: ___/26

19

PROXIMAL

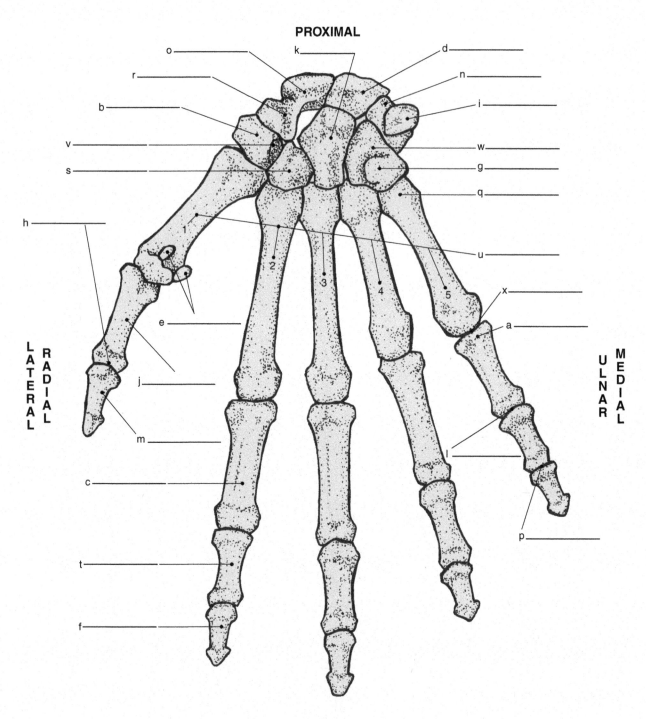

DISTAL

1. Base of metacarpal	7. Hamate	13. Middle phalanx of finger	19. Scaphoid tubercle
2. Base of phalanx	8. Hook of hamate	14. Pisiform	20. Sesamoid bones
3. Capitate	9. Interphalangeal joint	15. Proximal interphalangeal joint	21. Trapezium
4. Distal interphalangeal joint	10. Lunate	16. Proximal phalanx of finger	22. Trapezoid
5. Distal phalanx of finger	11. Metacarpals	17. Proximal phalanx of thumb	23. Triquetrum
6. Distal phalanx of thumb	12. Metacarpophalangeal joint	18. Scaphoid	24. Tubercle of trapezium

Score: ___/24

FILL IN THE BLANK

Fill in the blank with the answer that best completes each question or statement.

1. What bone is located in the thigh? _____

2. What bone is located in the arm? _____

3. What bones are located in the leg? _____

4. What bones are located in the forearm? _____

5. There are _____ cervical vertebrae.

6. The shoulder girdle is composed of the _____ and _____ bones.

7. There are _____ metacarpals in each hand.

8. There are _____ phalanges in each hand.

9. The _____ bones are located between the forearm and hand.

10. The _____ bones are located between the tibia and metatarsals.

11. How many ribs on each side attach into the sternum? _____

12. There are _____ tarsals in each foot.

13. Approximately how many bones are there in the adult human body? _____

14. _____ is the plural form of vertebra.

15. The singular form of phalanges is _____.

Score: ___/15

KNOW YOUR BONES

For each of the following questions, state whether the bone is axial or appendicular. Write your answer in the space provided.

1. Humerus: _____

2. Pelvic: _____

3. Carpal: _____

4. Vertebra: _____

5. Sternum: _____

6. Phalanx: _____

7. Radius: _____

8. Rib: _____

9. Tibia: _____

10. Cranial: _____

CROSSWORD PUZZLE

Use the clues to complete the crossword puzzle.

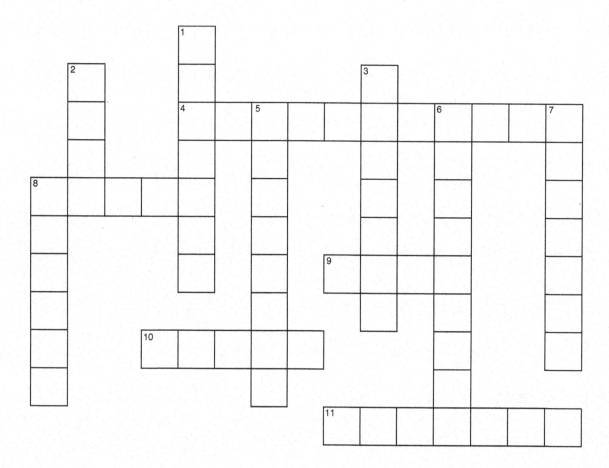

ACROSS

4 Distal to carpals
8 Distal to pelvic bone
9 Medial bone of forearm
10 Bone of leg
11 Ankle bones

DOWN

1 Proximal to radius
2 Number of vertebrae in sacrum
3 Wrist bones
5 Superior to lumbar vertebrae
6 Distal to metatarsals
7 Bone of shoulder joint
8 Lateral to tibia

COLORING & LABELING

Use crayons or felt-tipped markers to color the bones and bony landmarks. Use the word banks to fill in the numbers that correspond to the names of the bones and bony landmarks in the blanks provided.

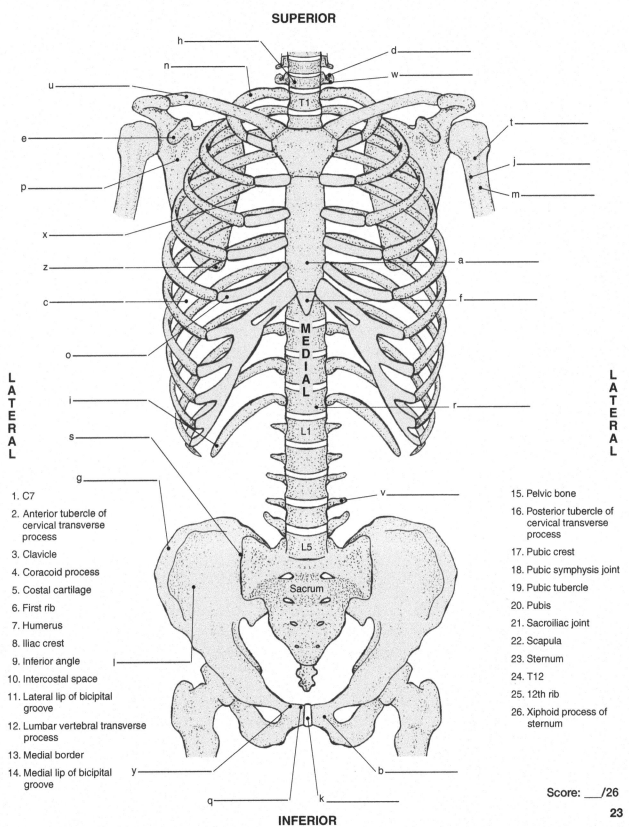

1. C7
2. Anterior tubercle of cervical transverse process
3. Clavicle
4. Coracoid process
5. Costal cartilage
6. First rib
7. Humerus
8. Iliac crest
9. Inferior angle
10. Intercostal space
11. Lateral lip of bicipital groove
12. Lumbar vertebral transverse process
13. Medial border
14. Medial lip of bicipital groove

15. Pelvic bone
16. Posterior tubercle of cervical transverse process
17. Pubic crest
18. Pubic symphysis joint
19. Pubic tubercle
20. Pubis
21. Sacroiliac joint
22. Scapula
23. Sternum
24. T12
25. 12th rib
26. Xiphoid process of sternum

Score: ___/26

23

SUPERIOR

LATERAL

LATERAL

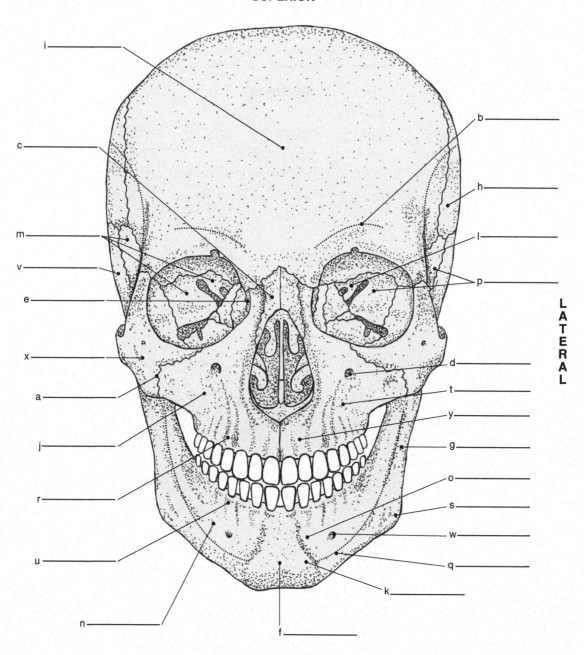

i

c

m

v

e

x

a

j

r

u

n

b

h

l

p

d

t

y

g

o

s

w

q

k

f

INFERIOR

1. Alveolar process
2. Alveolar process
3. Angle of mandible
4. Canine fossa
5. Frontal bone
6. Greater wing of sphenoid
7. Incisive fossa

8. Incisive fossa
9. Infraorbital foramen
10. Lacrimal bone
11. Lesser wing of sphenoid
12. Mandible
13. Maxilla

14. Mental foramen
15. Mental tubercle
16. Nasal bone
17. Oblique line
18. Ramus
19. Sphenoid bone

20. Superciliary arch
21. Symphysis menti
22. Temporal bone
23. Temporal fossa (within dotted line)
24. Zygomatic bone
25. Zygomaticomaxillary suture

Score: ___/25

24

PROXIMAL

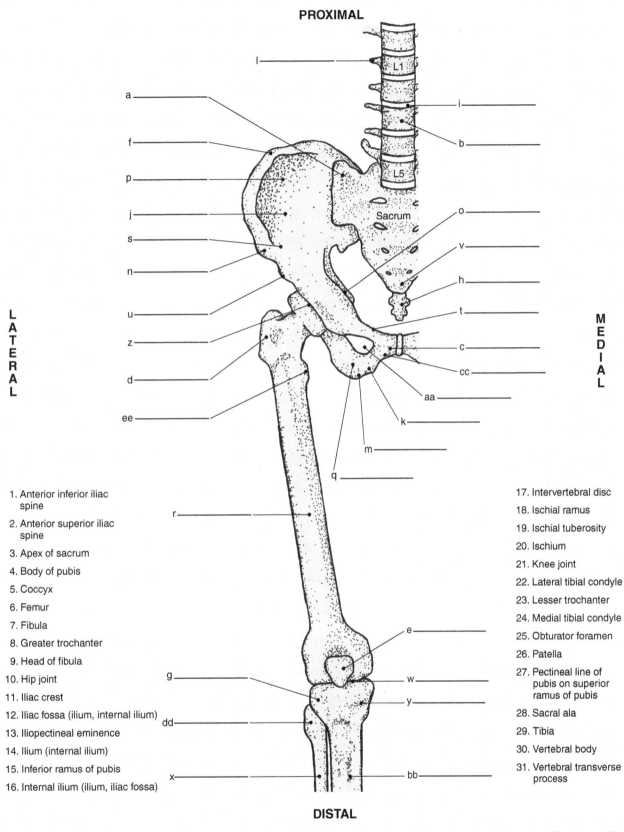

L1

L5

Sacrum

l

a

f

p

j

s

n

u

z

d

ee

i

b

o

v

h

t

c

cc

aa

k

m

q

r

e

g

w

y

dd

x

bb

L A T E R A L

M E D I A L

1. Anterior inferior iliac spine
2. Anterior superior iliac spine
3. Apex of sacrum
4. Body of pubis
5. Coccyx
6. Femur
7. Fibula
8. Greater trochanter
9. Head of fibula
10. Hip joint
11. Iliac crest
12. Iliac fossa (ilium, internal ilium)
13. Iliopectineal eminence
14. Ilium (internal ilium)
15. Inferior ramus of pubis
16. Internal ilium (ilium, iliac fossa)

17. Intervertebral disc
18. Ischial ramus
19. Ischial tuberosity
20. Ischium
21. Knee joint
22. Lateral tibial condyle
23. Lesser trochanter
24. Medial tibial condyle
25. Obturator foramen
26. Patella
27. Pectineal line of pubis on superior ramus of pubis
28. Sacral ala
29. Tibia
30. Vertebral body
31. Vertebral transverse process

DISTAL

Score: ___/31

25

PROXIMAL

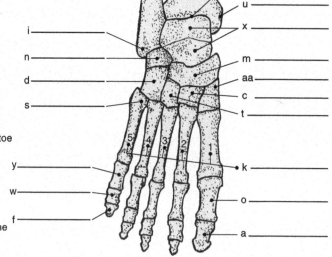

q

z

g

l

v

b

h

p

e

r

LATERAL

MEDIAL

j

u

x

i

n

d

s

m

aa

c

t

5 4 3 2 1

y

w

f

k

o

a

DISTAL

1. 1st cuneiform
2. 2nd cuneiform
3. 3rd cuneiform
4. Ankle joint
5. Base of metatarsal
6. Calcaneus
7. Cuboid
8. Distal phalanx of big toe
9. Distal phalanx of toe
10. Femur
11. Fibula
12. Head of fibula
13. Interosseus membrane
14. Knee joint

15. Lateral condyle of femur
16. Lateral condyle of tibia
17. Lateral malleolus
18. Lateral supracondylar line
19. Medial condyle of femur
20. Medial malleolus
21. Metatarsals
22. Middle phalanx of toe
23. Navicular
24. Proximal phalanx of big toe
25. Proximal phalanx of toe
26. Talus
27. Tibia

Score: ___/27

PROXIMAL

L A T E R A L

M E D I A L

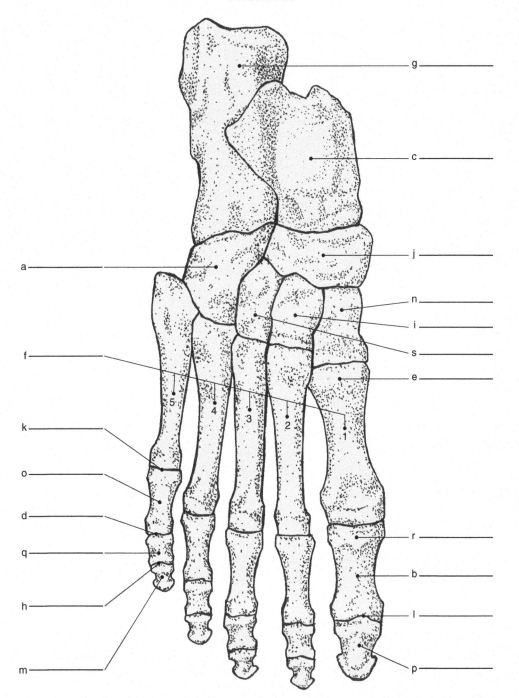

DISTAL

1. 1st cuneiform	6. Calcaneus	11. Interphalangeal (IP) joint	16. Proximal interphalangeal (PIP) joint
2. 2nd cuneiform	7. Cuboid	12. Metatarsals	17. Proximal phalanx of big toe
3. 3rd cuneiform	8. Distal interphalangeal (DIP) joint	13. Metatarsophalangeal (MTP) joint	18. Proximal phalanx of toe
4. Base of metatarsal	9. Distal phalanx of big toe	14. Middle phalanx of toe	19. Talus
5. Base of phalanx	10. Distal phalanx of toe	15. Navicular	

Score: ___/19

27

MATCHING

Match the joint type on the left with the proper definition on the right. Write the letter of your answer in the space provided. Each choice will be used only once.

Joint type

_____ 1. Uniaxial

_____ 2. Biaxial

_____ 3. Nonaxial

_____ 4. Synarthrotic

_____ 5. Diarthrotic

_____ 6. Amphiarthrotic

_____ 7. Fibrous

_____ 8. Cartilaginous

_____ 9. Triaxial

_____ 10. Synovial

Definition

a. United by fibrous tissue
b. United by fibrocartilage
c. United by thin fibrous capsule that is lined by synovial membrane
d. Permits very little motion
e. Permits limited to moderate motion
f. Permits a great deal of motion
g. Permits motion around one axis
h. Permits motion around two axes
i. Permits motion around three axes
j. Permits only linear gliding motion

Score: ___/10

TRUE OR FALSE

Write T on the line if the statement is true or F if the statement is false.

1. _____ Pivot and hinge joints are biaxial.

2. _____ Ball-and-socket joints are triaxial.

3. _____ Only synovial joints have a joint cavity.

4. _____ Fibrous joints are usually synarthrotic.

5. _____ Synovial joints are usually amphiarthrotic.

Score: ___/5

FILL IN THE BLANK

Fill in the blank with the answer that best completes each question or statement.

1. What is the structural definition of a joint? _____

2. What are the three structural classifications of joints? _____, _____, &

   _____

3. What is the functional definition of a joint? _____

4. What are the three functional classifications of joints? _____, _____, &

_____

5. What are the four axial motion classifications of joints? _____, _____,

_____, & _____

MULTIPLE CHOICE

Circle the letter of the best answer to the question.

1. Which of the following are biaxial joints?
   a. Condyloid, ball-and-socket
   b. Saddle, condyloid
   c. Hinge, saddle
   d. All of the above

2. Which of the following joints are uniaxial?
   a. Hinge and saddle
   b. Saddle and condyloid
   c. Ball-and-socket
   d. Hinge and pivot

3. Which of the following joints permits only rotation?
   a. Pivot
   b. Hinge
   c. Ball-and-socket
   d. Saddle

4. Which of the following joint types permit the most motion?
   a. Synarthrotic
   b. Amphiarthrotic
   c. Synovial
   d. Fibrous

5. In what plane(s) does a pivot joint allow motion?
   a. Frontal and sagittal
   b. Transverse only
   c. Transverse and sagittal
   d. Sagittal only

Use the clues to complete the crossword puzzle.

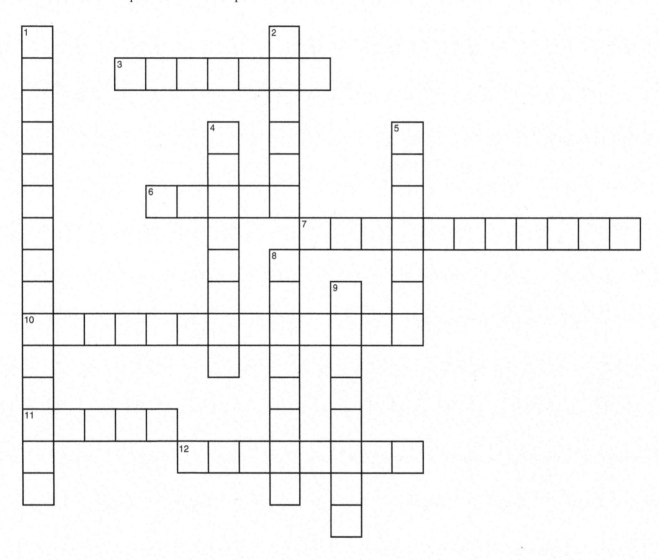

ACROSS

3 Motion around two axes
6 Motion only in sagittal plane
7 Most movable type of joint
10 Amphiarthrotic
11 Atlantoaxial joint
12 Motion around three axes

DOWN

1 Saddle joint of thumb
2 Each bone of joint has
  convex and concave shape
4 Diarthrotic
5 Synarthrotic
8 Motion around one axis
9 Linear gliding motion only

Score: ___/12

3 How Muscles Function

Use crayons or felt-tipped markers to color the muscle actions.

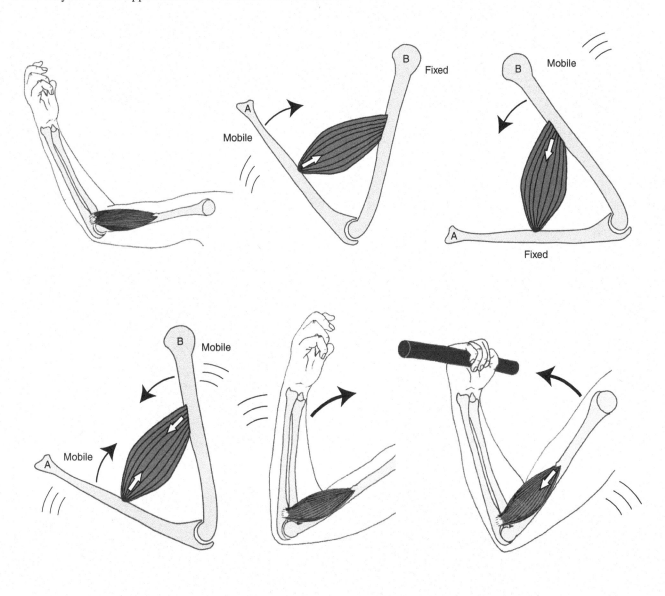

31

Use crayons or felt-tipped markers to color the muscles. Use the word bank to fill in the names of the muscles in the blanks provided.

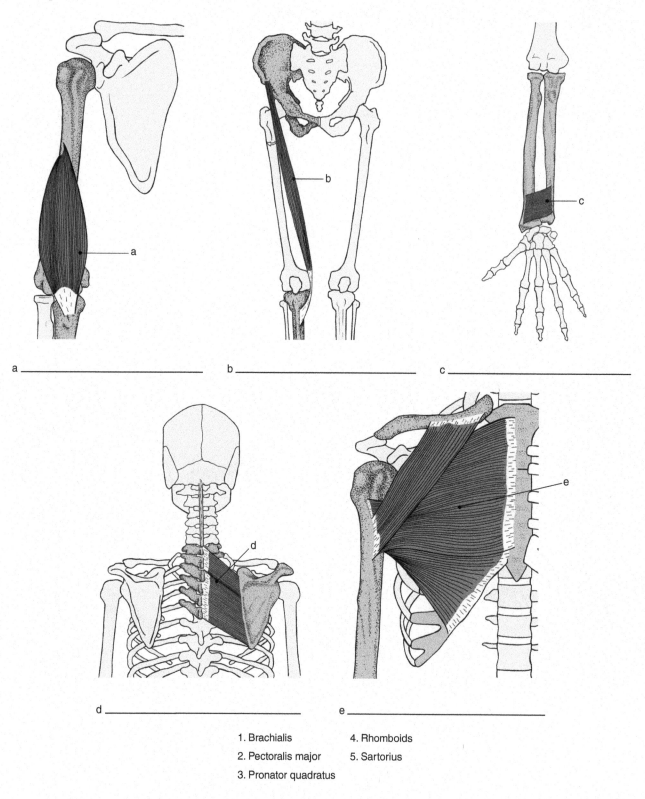

a _____

b _____

c _____

d _____

e _____

1. Brachialis   4. Rhomboids
2. Pectoralis major   5. Sartorius
3. Pronator quadratus

Score: ___/5

Place the appropriate letter from column 2 (Length of the muscle) and from column 3 (Strength of contraction) into the blanks next to the type of contraction in column 1. Each choice should be used only once.

Type of contraction	Length of muscle	Strength of contraction
___ ___ 1. Concentric	a. Lengthening	d. Equal to resistance force
___ ___ 2. Eccentric	b. Stays the same length	e. Greater than resistance force
___ ___ 3. Isometric	c. Shortening	f. Less than resistance force

Score: ___/3

LINE MATCHING

Arrange the *5-Step Approach to Learning Muscles* by drawing a line from the step number to the appropriate step description.

Description of Step	Step Number
1. Look at name	Step 1
2. Memorize specific attachments	Step 2
3. Learn general location	Step 3
4. Figure out actions	Step 4
5. Look at relationship to other structures	Step 5

Score: ___/5

CONTRACTIONS

For each of the following scenarios, state whether the muscle listed in parentheses is contracting concentrically, eccentrically, isometrically, or is relaxed.

1. Raising a weight doing a biceps curl (elbow joint flexors). _____

2. Raising a weight doing a biceps curl (elbow joint extensors). _____

3. Slowly lowering a weight doing a biceps curl (elbow joint flexors). _____

4. Slowly lowering a weight doing a biceps curl (elbow joint extensors). _____

5. Holding a weight in a static position halfway between full elbow joint flexion and full elbow joint extension when doing a biceps curl (elbow joint flexors). _____

6. Holding a weight in a static position halfway between full elbow joint flexion and full elbow joint extension when doing a biceps curl (elbow joint extensors). _____

7. Standing in anatomic position and raising the arm into abduction (glenohumeral joint abductors). _____

8. Standing in anatomic position and raising the arm into abduction (glenohumeral joint adductors). _____

9. Standing in anatomic position and slowly lowering the arm into adduction from an abducted position (glenohumeral joint abductors). _____

10. Standing in anatomic position and slowly lowering the arm into adduction from an abducted position (glenohumeral joint adductors). _____

11. Holding the arm in a static position halfway between full glenohumeral joint abduction and full glenohumeral joint adduction (glenohumeral joint abductors). _____

12. Holding the arm in a static position halfway between full glenohumeral joint abduction and full glenohumeral joint adduction (glenohumeral joint adductors). _____

13. In the preceding questions, was there a relationship between how muscle groups worked when the motion was moving up away from the ground or down toward the ground? If so, what was it?

_____

_____

_____

Score: ___/13

ACTIONS

For each of the following scenarios, state whether the concentric contraction is a **standard** action or a **reverse** action.

1. Flexion of the arm at the elbow joint. _____

2. Flexion of the forearm at the elbow joint. _____

3. Biceps curl. _____

4. Chin up (at the elbow joint). _____

5. The distal attachment moves toward the proximal one. _____

6. The proximal attachment moves toward the distal one. _____

7. Standing up from a seated position (at the knee joint). _____

8. Origin moves toward the insertion. _____

9. Insertion moves toward the origin. _____

10. Reaching forward with the thigh to take a step when walking (at the hip joint). _____

Score: ___/10

TRUE OR FALSE

Write a T on the line if the statement is true or F if the statement is false.

1. _____ When a muscle contracts, it can choose to pull only one of its attachments.

2. _____ The origin of a muscle always stays fixed.

3. _____ The origin of a muscle is usually the proximal attachment.

4. _____ A muscle cell is a muscle fiber.

5. _____ The major purpose of a muscle's tendon is to transmit the pulling force of the muscle onto its attachment.

Score: ___/5

FILL IN THE BLANK

Fill in the blank with the answer that best completes each question or statement.

1. The essence of muscle function is that muscles create _____.

2. When do reverse actions usually occur in the lower extremity? _____

3. Give an everyday example of a reverse action in the upper extremity.

   _____

4. What are the three fibrous fascial layers of a muscle?

   _____

5. What type of contraction occurs when myosin heads succeed in pulling actin filaments toward the center of the sarcomere? _____

6. The two types of muscle fiber architecture are _____ and _____.

7. What three questions must be asked and answered in Step 3 of the *5-Step Approach to Learning Muscles*?

   _____

   _____

   _____

8. It can be helpful to look at a muscle as either crossing a joint _____ or _____.

9. All muscles that can flex the arm at the glenohumeral joint are said to be members of the same

   _____.

10. What simple tool can be used to simulate a muscle's pull and thereby learn its actions? _____

Score: ___/10

35

Circle the letter of the best answer to the question.

1. When a muscle contracts, it
   a. always shortens
   b. always lengthens
   c. always stays the same length
   d. None of the above

2. Which of the following is true regarding the origin of a muscle?
   a. It always stays fixed.
   b. It always moves.
   c. It is usually the proximal attachment.
   d. It is usually the distal attachment.

3. What term describes a tendon that is broad and flat in shape?
   a. Endomysium
   b. Sarcomere
   c. Aponeurosis
   d. Pennate

4. Which of the following is true regarding sarcomeres?
   a. Actin filaments are thin.
   b. Myosin filaments have heads.
   c. Z-lines are the borders.
   d. All of the above

5. Which of the following defines a muscle contraction?
   a. The muscle shortens.
   b. Myosin heads pull on actin filaments.
   c. A concentric contraction
   d. All of the above

Score: ___/5

Chapter 3 *How Muscles Function*

Use the clues to complete the crossword puzzle.

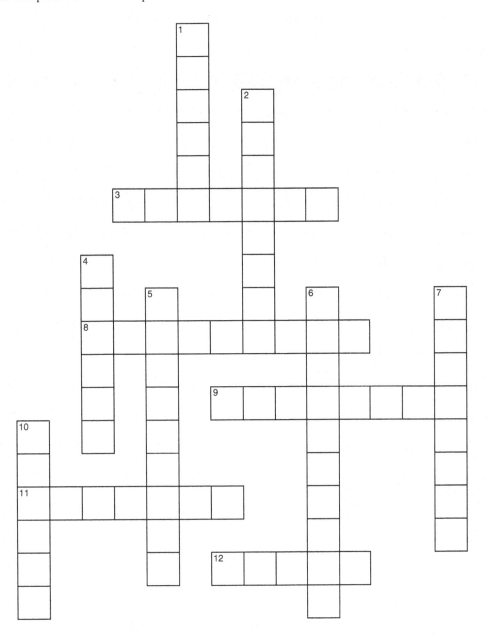

ACROSS

3 Type of muscle fiber architecture
8 Distal attachment
9 Group of muscle fibers
11 Proximal attachment moves
12 Attaches to Z-line

DOWN

1 Actin and _____
2 Sliding _____ mechanism
4 Proximal attachment
5 Stabilizer contraction
6 Shortening contraction
7 When a muscle contracts,
  it _____ to shorten
10 Z-line of sarcomere

Score: ___/12

HOW TO PALPATE

KNOW YOUR MUSCLES

Use your textbook to locate, palpate, and identify the muscles in the figures. Fill in the blank with the name of the muscle being palpated, and use your own words to write a brief description of the palpation.

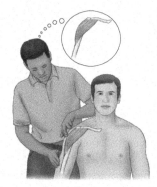

a. _____

_____

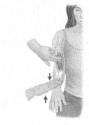

b. _____

_____

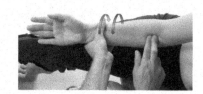

c. _____

_____

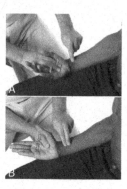

d. _____

_____

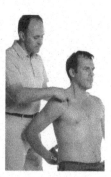

e. _____

_____

Score: ___/10

MATCHING

Match the muscle from the right column to its description in the left column. Write your answer in the space provided. Each choice will be used only once.

1. _____ Engaged and palpated when the forearm pronates.

2. _____ Engaged and palpated when the thigh flexes and medially rotates.

3. _____ Engaged and palpated when the neck contralaterally rotates.

4. _____ Palpated by reciprocally inhibiting the biceps brachii.

5. _____ Palpated by reciprocally inhibiting the upper trapezius.

6. _____ Located lateral to sacrum, halfway between the posterior superior iliac spine (PSIS) and the apex of sacrum.

7. _____ Engaged and palpated with the hand located in the small of back.

8. _____ Engaged and palpated with dorsiflexion and inversion.

9. _____ Sink slowly toward spine to palpate this muscle.

10. _____ Engaged and palpated with flexion of the distal phalanx of the thumb.

a. Psoas major
b. Brachialis
c. Tensor fasciae latae
d. Tibialis anterior
e. Rhomboids
f. Sternocleidomastoid
g. Flexor pollicis longus
h. Pronator teres
i. Piriformis
j. Levator scapulae

Score: ___/10

TRUE OR FALSE

Write a T on the line if the statement is true or F if the statement is false.

1. _____ The word *palpation* comes from the Latin word meaning "to touch."

2. _____ It is important to "feel" with our brains as well as our fingers.

3. _____ If the client moves a body part that is not part of the palpation protocol, it is best for the therapist to manually resist that movement.

4. _____ When adding resistance, it is important that the therapist does not cross any additional joints with the placement of the stabilization (resistance) hand.

5. _____ It is best to first find the target muscle in the most difficult place possible.

6. _____ Light pressure is always better when palpating.

7. _____ When palpating the bony attachment of a muscle, it is usually best for the muscle to be relaxed.

Score: ___/7

FILL IN THE BLANK

Fill in the blank with the answer that best completes each question or statement.

1. What are the first two guidelines of palpation?

_____

_____

2. When should we be palpating? _____

3. What are the two objectives of palpation? _____

4. What are the primary assessment tools of the manual therapist?

_____

5. What are the two best ways to palpate deep musculature?

_____

Score: ___/5

MULTIPLE CHOICE

General Palpation
Circle the letter of the best answer to the question.

1. Which aspect of the target muscle is important to palpate?
   a. Its belly
   b. Its proximal attachment
   c. Its distal attachment
   d. All of the above

2. Which of the following best describes how assessment and treatment should be carried out?
   a. All assessment should be done first, then treatment.
   b. All treatment should be done first, then assessment.
   c. We assess while we treat.
   d. None of the above

3. Why is it helpful to ask the client to engage and contract the target muscle being palpated?
   a. It will be soft amidst adjacent soft tissues.
   b. It will be soft amidst adjacent hard tissues.
   c. It will be hard amidst adjacent soft tissues.
   d. It will be hard amidst adjacent hard tissues.

4. What knowledge is most necessary to have an isolated contraction of the target muscle?
   a. The attachments of the target muscle only
   b. The actions of the target muscle only
   c. The attachments of the target and adjacent musculature
   d. The actions of the target and adjacent musculature

5. For which of the following muscles is it most important to look before you palpate?
   a. Flexor carpi radialis
   b. Serratus posterior superior
   c. Multifidus
   d. Supinator

6. Once the target muscle has been located, what is the best way to palpate it?
   a. Glide along it longitudinally.
   b. Press into it with static compression.
   c. Strum perpendicularly.
   d. Palpate across it diagonally to its direction of fibers.

7. How is it usually best for the client to engage the target muscle during the palpation protocol?
   a. Hold a sustained contraction.
   b. Alternately contract and relax the target muscle.
   c. Keep the target muscle relaxed.
   d. None of the above. It is does matter how the client engages the target muscle.

8. Which of the following are coupled actions that would best engage the pectoralis minor?
   a. Extension of the arm/downward rotation of the scapula
   b. Flexion of the arm/upward rotation of the scapula
   c. Extension of the arm/upward rotation of the scapula
   d. Flexion of the arm/downward rotation of the scapula

9. During which of the following muscle palpations is it most important for the client to breathe?
   a. Flexor carpi radialis
   b. Psoas major
   c. Rectus femoris
   d. Upper trapezius

10. Which of the following is the best example of using one muscle as a landmark to find another?
   a. Flexor carpi ulnaris for pronator teres
   b. Serratus posterior superior for serratus anterior
   c. Sternocleidomastoid for scalenes
   d. Tibialis anterior for tibialis posterior

Score: ___/10

MULTIPLE CHOICE

Isolated Contraction

Circle the letter of the best answer to the question.

1. Which of the following actions would best allow the therapist to palpate the flexor carpi radialis and discern it from the palmaris longus?
   a. Flexion of the hand at the wrist joint
   b. Ulnar deviation of the hand at the wrist joint
   c. Radial deviation of the hand at the wrist joint
   d. Flexion of the forearm at the elbow joint

2. Which of the following actions would best allow the therapist to palpate the fibularis longus and discern it from the extensor digitorum longus?
   a. Eversion of the foot
   b. Plantarflexion of the foot
   c. Flexion of the leg
   d. Inversion of the foot

3. Which of the following actions would best allow the therapist to palpate the rectus femoris and discern it from the vastus lateralis?
   a. Flexion of the hip joint
   b. Extension of the hip joint
   c. Flexion of the knee joint
   d. Extension of the knee joint

41

4. Which of the following actions would best allow the therapist to palpate the right upper trapezius and discern it from the right splenius capitis?
   a. Extension of the neck
   b. Flexion of the neck
   c. Left rotation of the neck
   d. Right lateral flexion of the neck

5. Which of the following actions would best allow the therapist to palpate the pronator teres and discern it from the flexor carpi radialis?
   a. Flexion of the elbow joint
   b. Flexion of the wrist joint
   c. Pronation of the forearm
   d. Ulnar deviation of the wrist joint

Score: ___/5

MULTIPLE CHOICE

Resistance

Circle the letter of the best answer to the question.

1. In what location should resistance be added when palpating the pronator teres?
   a. Distal forearm
   b. Proximal arm
   c. Palm of hand
   d. Fingers

2. In what location should resistance be added when palpating the tensor fasciae latae?
   a. Pelvis
   b. Thigh
   c. Leg
   d. Foot

3. In what location should resistance be added when palpating the brachioradialis?
   a. Arm
   b. Hand
   c. Forearm
   d. Shoulder girdle

4. In what location should resistance be added when palpating the flexor pollicis longus?
   a. Distal forearm
   b. Metacarpal of thumb
   c. Proximal phalanx of thumb
   d. Distal phalanx of thumb

5. In what location should resistance be added when palpating the gluteus maximus?
   a. Pelvis
   b. Thigh
   c. Leg
   d. Foot

Score: ___/5

CROSSWORD PUZZLE

Use the clues to complete the crossword puzzle.

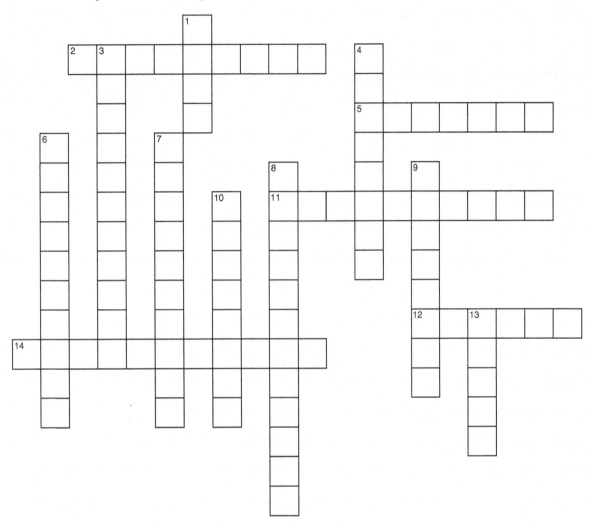

ACROSS

2 Latin for "to touch."
5 For scapular rotators, use _____ actions.
11 Reciprocal _____.
12 Locate and then _____.
14 _____ contract and relax.

DOWN

1 Always follow the muscle using _____ steps.
3 Use _____ pressure.
4 For the _____ client, place their hand over ours.
6 Think _____ to choose the best action.
7 When adding _____, never cross a joint that does not need to be crossed.
8 Fluid interplay between assessment and treatment (2 words).
9 Palpatory _____.
10 The best contraction for palpation.
13 _____ perpendicularly.

Score: ___/14

5 | Bony Palpation

COLORING & LABELING

Use crayons or felt-tipped markers to color the bones and bony landmarks. Use the word banks to fill in the numbers that correspond to the names of the bones and bony landmarks in the blanks provided.

ANTEROMEDIAL VIEW

1. Acromion process
2. Clavicle
3. Coracoid process
4. Head of humerus
5. Sternum
6. Suprasternal notch

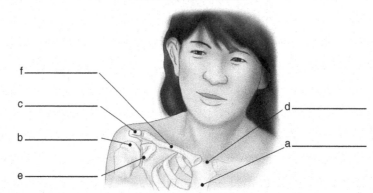

f _____
c _____
b _____
e _____
d _____
a _____

Score: __/6

POSTEROLATERAL VIEW

1. Acromion process
2. Inferior angle
3. Infraspinous fossa
4. Lateral border
5. Medial border
6. Spine of scapula
7. Superior angle
8. Superior border
9. Supraspinous fossa

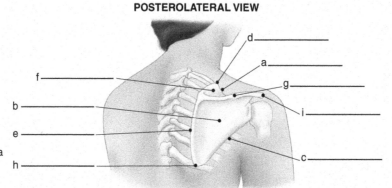

f _____
b _____
e _____
h _____
d _____
a _____
g _____
i _____
c _____

Score: __/9

LATERAL VIEW

1. Dorsal tubercle of radius
2. Saddle joint
3. Scaphoid
4. Styloid process of radius
5. Styloid process of ulna
6. Trapezium

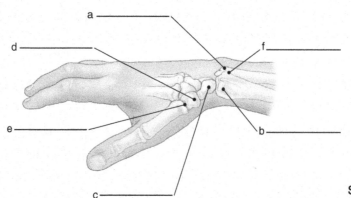

a _____
d _____
e _____
c _____
f _____
b _____

Score: __/6

ANTERIOR (PALMAR) VIEW

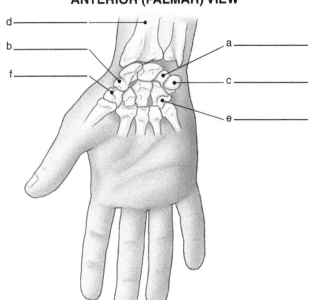

1. Hook of hamate
2. Pisiform
3. Radius
4. Triquetrum
5. Tubercle of scaphoid
6. Tubercle of trapezium

Score: __/6

INFEROLATERAL VIEW

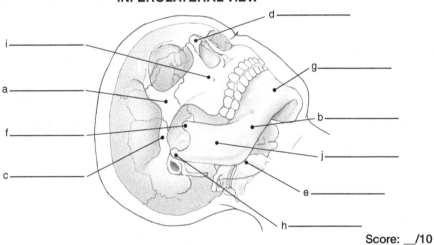

1. Angle
2. Body of mandible
3. Condyle
4. Coronoid process
5. Mandible
6. Maxilla
7. Nasal bone
8. Ramus
9. Zygomatic arch of the temporal bone
10. Zygomatic bone

Score: __/10

LATERAL VIEW

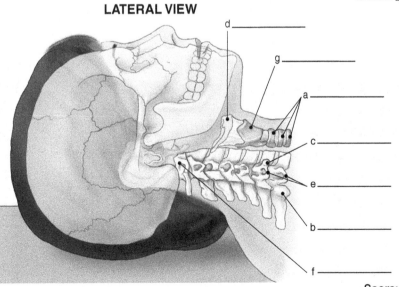

1. C1
2. C7
3. Carotid tubercle
4. Cricoid cartilages
5. Hyoid bone
6. Thyroid cartilage
7. Transverse processes

Score: __/7

45

SUPEROLATERAL VIEW

1. 11th rib
2. 1st rib
3. 2nd intercostal space
4. 7th rib
5. Body of sternum
6. Clavicle
7. Costal cartilage of 3rd rib
8. Iliac crest
9. Manubrium
10. Suprasternal notch
11. Xiphoid process

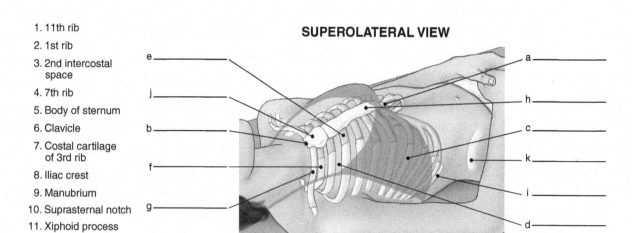

Score: __/11

POSTEROLATERAL VIEW

1. 5th rib
2. 9th rib
3. Lamina of T7
4. SP of T1
5. SP of T6
6. TP of T6

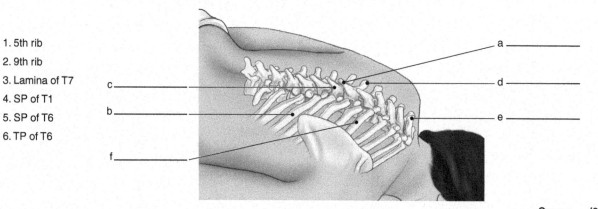

Score: __/6

OBLIQUE VIEW

1. 2nd sacral tubercle
2. Coccyx
3. Iliac crest
4. Ischial tuberosity
5. Posterior superior iliac spine
6. Sacrococcygeal joint
7. Sacrum

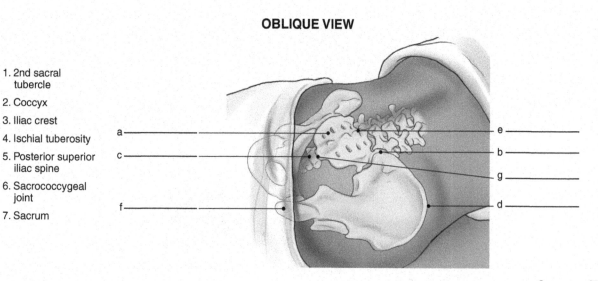

Score: __/7

ANTEROLATERAL VIEW

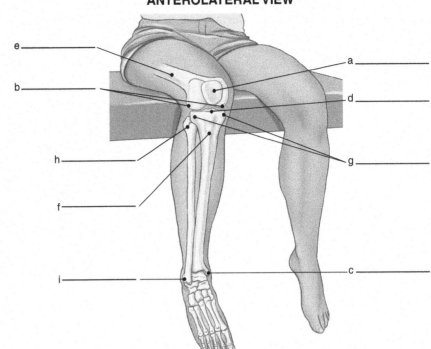

e ——————
b ——————
h ——————
f ——————

a ——————————
d ——————————
g ——————————
c ——————————
i ——————

1. Femoral condyles
2. Femur
3. Head of fibula
4. Knee joint
5. Lateral malleolus
6. Medial malleolus
7. Patella
8. Tibial condyles
9. Tibial tuberosity

Score: __/9

MEDIAL VIEW

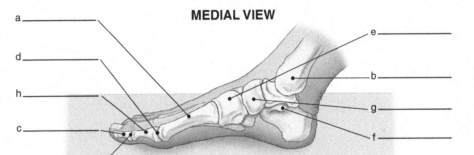

1. 1st cuneiform
2. 1st metatarsal
3. Distal phalanx
4. Interphalangeal joint
5. Medial malleolus of tibia
6. Metatarsophalangeal joint
7. Navicular tuberosity
8. Proximal phalanx
9. Sustentaculum tali of calcaneus

a ——————
d ——————
h ——————
c ——————
i ——————

e ——————————
b ——————————
g ——————————
f ——————————

Score: __/9

PLANTAR VIEW

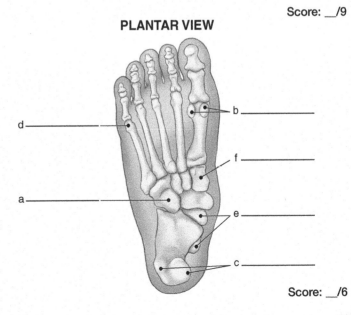

1. 1st cuneiform
2. 5th metatarsal head
3. Calcaneal tuberosity
4. Cuboid
5. Sesamoid bones overlying 1st metatarsal head
6. Talus

d ——————
a ——————

b ——————————
f ——————————
e ——————————
c ——————————

Score: __/6

47

Use your textbook to locate, palpate, and identify the bone or bony landmark in the figures. Fill in the blank with the name of the bone or bony landmark being palpated, and use your own words to write a brief description of the palpation.

1.

ANTEROMEDIAL VIEW

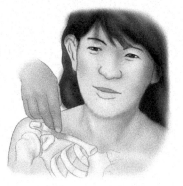

_____

_____

2.

POSTEROLATERAL VIEW

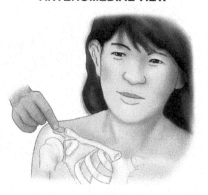

_____

_____

3.

ANTEROMEDIAL VIEW

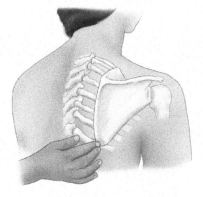

_____

_____

Chapter **5** **Bony Palpation**

4.

POSTERIOR VIEW

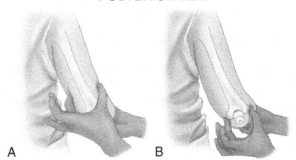

A   B

_____

_____

5.

LATERAL VIEW

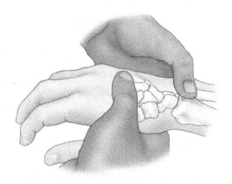

_____

_____

6.

LATERAL VIEW

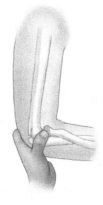

_____

_____

Chapter **5** **Bony Palpation**

7.

POSTEROLATERAL VIEW

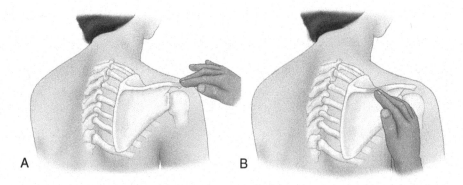

A   B

_____

_____

8.

ANTEROMEDIAL VIEW

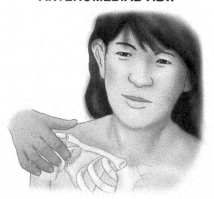

_____

_____

Score: __/16

TRUE OR FALSE

Write a T on the line if the statement is true or F if the statement is false.

1. _____ The root of the spine of the scapula is palpated where the spine meets the lateral border of the scapula.

2. _____ The styloid process of the ulna is palpated at the distal end of the anterior ulna.

3. _____ The trapezium is the most prominent carpal that can be palpated on the anterior radial side of the wrist.

4. _____ The medial and lateral epicondyles of the humerus are best palpated with the client's elbow joint flexed approximately 90 degrees.

Score: __/4

FILL IN THE BLANK

Fill in the blank with the answer that best completes each question.

1. What landmark is palpated anteriorly, directly inferior to the lateral clavicle? _____.

2. What landmark is palpated at the inferior aspect of the medial border of the scapula? _____.

3. What landmark is palpated immediately medial to the bicipital groove of the humerus? _____.

4. What landmark is palpated immediately distal to the lateral epicondyle of the humerus? _____.

Score: __/4

MULTIPLE CHOICE

Circle the letter of the best answer to the question.

1. What carpal bone is palpated just distal to the pisiform?
   a. Triquetrum
   b. Hamate
   c. Scaphoid
   d. Trapezium

2. Which of the following is true regarding the shape of the clavicle anteriorly?
   a. The entire clavicle is convex.
   b. The entire clavicle is concave.
   c. The medial clavicle is convex; the lateral clavicle is concave.
   d. The medial clavicle is concave; the lateral clavicle is convex.

3. In what direction does the tip of the coracoid process point?
   a. Medially
   b. Laterally
   c. Superiorly
   d. Inferiorly

4. The palpation of what bony landmarks is facilitated by passive lateral and medial rotation of the humerus?
   a. Medial and lateral condyles of humerus
   b. Radial head and ulnar olecranon process
   c. Medial condyle and lesser tubercle of humerus
   d. Greater and lesser tubercles of humerus

Score: __/4

CROSSWORD PUZZLE

Use the clues to complete the crossword puzzle.

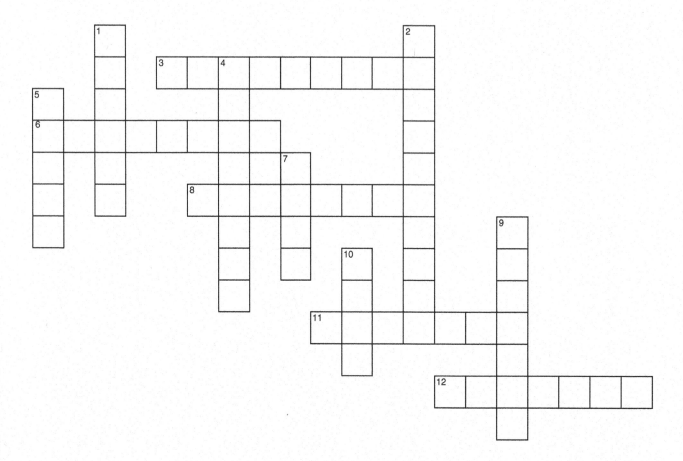

ACROSS

3 Groove between greater and lesser tubercles.
6 Prominent carpal on ulnar side.
8 Tip of shoulder.
11 Infraglenoid tubercle at the top of this scapular border.
12 Engage this muscle for infraglenoid tubercle palpation.

DOWN

1 Also known as Lister's tubercle.
2 Next to olecranon process (2 words).
4 Bony landmark deep to pectoralis major.
5 Posterior continuation of acromion.
7 _____ of hamate.
9 Both radius and ulna have this structure.
10 Radial landmark palpated with alternating pronation and supination.

Score: __/12

KNOW YOUR BONES

Use your textbook to locate, palpate, and identify the bone or bony landmark in the figures. Fill in the blank with the name of the bone or bony landmark being palpated, and use your own words to write a brief description of the palpation.

1.

INFEROLATERAL VIEW

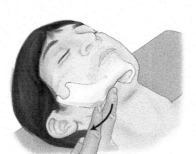

_____

_____

2.

LATERAL VIEW

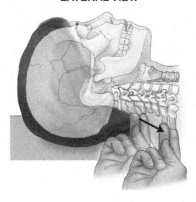

_____

_____

3.

LATERAL VIEW

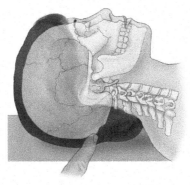

_____

_____

4.

SUPEROLATERAL VIEW

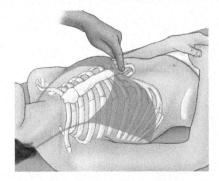

_____

_____

5.

LATERAL VIEW

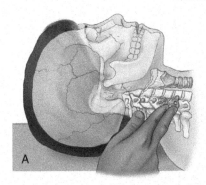 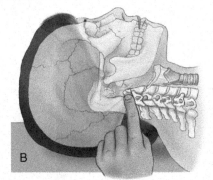

_____

_____

6.

LATERAL VIEW

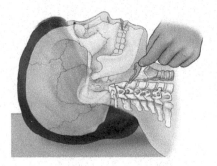

_____

_____

7.

LATERAL VIEW

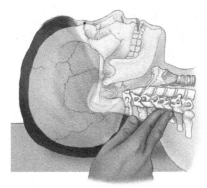

_____

_____

8.

INFEROLATERAL VIEW

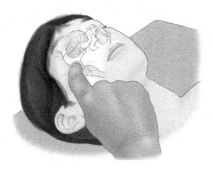

_____

_____

Score: __/16

TRUE OR FALSE

Write a T on the line if the statement is true or F if the statement is false.

1. _____ C2 is also known as the _vertebral prominens_.

2. _____ The external occipital protuberance can be palpated midline on the superior nuchal line of the occiput.

3. _____ The xiphoid process is the most inferior aspect of the sternum.

4. _____ To better palpate the condyle of the mandible, ask the client to open and close the mouth.

Score: __/4

FILL IN THE BLANK

Fill in the blank with the answer that best completes each question.

1. What name is given to the column of facets in the cervical spine?

   _____

2. What name is given to the anterior tubercle of the transverse process of C6?

   _____

3. The spinous processes of which two cervical vertebrae are most easily palpated?

   _____

4. What should we ask the client to do to facilitate palpation of the first rib?

   _____

Score: __/4

MULTIPLE CHOICE

Circle the letter of the best answer to the question.

1. What landmark is palpated immediately lateral to the spinous processes?
   a. Laminar groove
   b. Articular facet
   c. Transverse process
   d. Body

2. What rib is palpated directly anterior to the superior border of the upper trapezius?
   a. 1st
   b. 2nd
   c. 3rd
   d. 5th

3. What landmark is palpated immediately lateral to the laminar groove?
   a. Spinous process
   b. Transverse process
   c. Pedicle
   d. Facet

4. Relative to the mastoid process of the temporal bone, where is the transverse process of the atlas palpated?
   a. Posterior
   b. Superior
   c. Inferior
   d. Anterior

Score: __/4

CROSSWORD PUZZLE

Use the clues to complete the crossword puzzle.

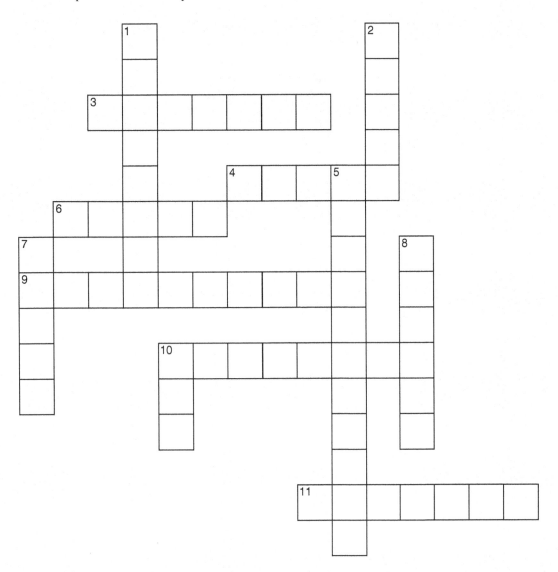

ACROSS

3 Suprasternal notch.
4 No articulation with another bone.
6 Zygomatic bone is the_____ bone.
9 Approximately 1 inch lateral to spinous process.
10 C1's version of a spinous process.
11 Groove located between spinous processes and facets.

DOWN

1 Number of costal cartilages that meet the sternum.
2 Two points.
5 Space between ribs.
7 Widest transverse process of cervical spine.
8 Articular processes.
10 Temporomandibular joint.

Score: __/12

Chapter 5 Bony Palpation

KNOW YOUR BONES

Use your textbook to locate, palpate, and identify the bone or bony landmark in the figures. Fill in the blank with the name of the bone or bony landmark being palpated, and use your own words to write a brief description of the palpation.

1.

PLANTAR VIEW

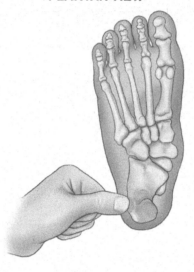

_____

_____

2.

ANTEROLATERAL VIEW

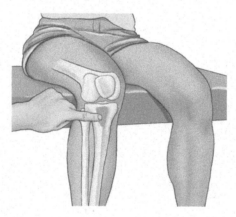

_____

_____

3.

MEDIAL VIEW

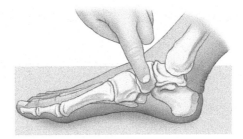

_____

_____

4.

INFEROLATERAL VIEW

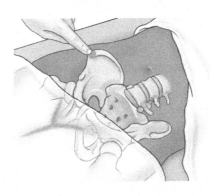

_____

_____

5.

INFEROLATERAL VIEW

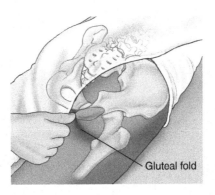

Gluteal fold

_____

_____

6.

ANTEROLATERAL VIEW

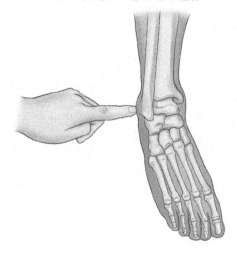

_____

_____

7.

SUPEROLATERAL VIEW

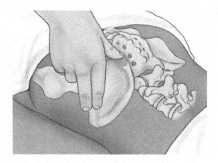

_____

_____

8.

DISTAL VIEW

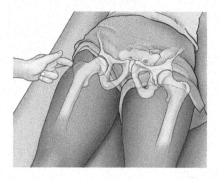

_____

_____

TRUE OR FALSE

Write a T on the line if the statement is true or F if the statement is false.

1. _____ The calcaneal tuberosity is palpated on the dorsal side of the foot.

2. _____ The greater trochanter is palpated in the proximal lateral thigh.

3. _____ Follow the psoas major to find the lesser trochanter of the femur.

4. _____ The tibial tuberosity is palpated approximately 1 to 2 inches distal to the patella.

Score:__/4

FILL IN THE BLANK

Fill in the blank with the answer that best completes each question.

1. What is the most anterior aspect of the iliac crest? _____

2. The _____ is the most distal aspect of the tibia.

3. What landmark can be palpated approximately 1 inch anterior to the sustentaculum tali of the calcaneus?

   _____

4. Due to the presence of the common fibular nerve, caution should be exercised when palpating the

   _____ .

Score: __/4

MULTIPLE CHOICE

Circle the letter of the best answer to the question.

1. In what direction is it best to palpate when locating the pubic tubercle?
   a. Inferior to superior
   b. Medial to lateral
   c. Lateral to medial
   d. Superior to inferior

2. What bony landmark is found by descending immediately inferior to the external occipital protuberance?
   a. Vertebral prominens
   b. C1 facet
   c. C2 laminar groove
   d. C2 spinous process

3. What aspect of the tibial shaft is superficial and easily palpable?
   a. Anteromedial
   b. Anterolateral
   c. Posteromedial
   d. Posterolateral

4. What bony landmark is palpated approximately 1 inch distal to the medial malleolus of the tibia?
   a. Navicular tuberosity
   b. Sustentaculum tali
   c. Cuboid bone
   d. Calcaneal tuberosity

Score: __/4

Use the clues to complete the crossword puzzle.

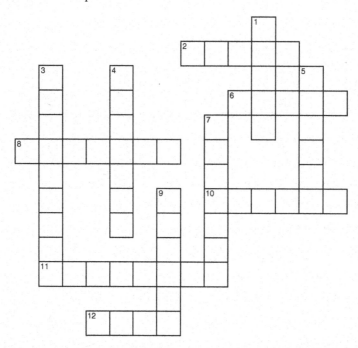

ACROSS

2 Palpate pubic tubercle with this side of hand.
6 The greater trochanter is located at the same level as this tubercle.
8 The ischial tuberosity is deep to this fold of tissue.
10 Medial trochanter.
11 Over first metatarsal head.
12 Proximal fibular landmark.

DOWN

1 Sustentaculum tali supports this bone.
3 Medial one for tibia; lateral one for fibula.
4 More distal malleolus.
5 The posterior superior iliac spine forms this.
7 Process of 5th metatarsal where it flares out.
9 Palpated immediately proximal to 5th metatarsal.

Score: __/12

CHAPTERS 1–5 SUMMARY REVIEW - MULTIPLE CHOICE

Circle the letter of the best answer to the question.

1. The _____ plane divides the body into left and right portions.
   a. Frontal
   b. Oblique
   c. Sagittal
   d. Transverse

2. Which of the following is a synovial uniaxial joint?
   a. Ball-in-socket
   b. Pivot
   c. Hinge
   d. Both B and C

3. The term _____ means "with center," and refers to a shortening contraction of a muscle.
   a. Eccentric
   b. Concentric
   c. Isometric
   d. Reverse action

4. What is the term that refers to a collective bundle of muscle fibers?
   a. Aponeurosis
   b. Sarcomere
   c. Myofibril
   d. Fascicle

5. Which of the following must be considered when developing an accurate client assessment?
   a. Visual observation
   b. History
   c. Client's response to treatment
   d. All of the above

6. When the client's contraction of the target muscle is not forceful enough, it might be necessary for the therapist to do which of the following?
   a. Add resistance.
   b. Remove resistance.
   c. Ask the client to alternate contraction and relaxation.
   d. None of the above

7. Which of the following is a neurologic reflex that causes inhibition of a muscle whenever an antagonist muscle is actively contracted?
   a. Coupled action
   b. Reciprocal inhibition
   c. Baby steps
   d. Motor pressure

8. If the client is ticklish, the therapist should…
   a. Close the eyes when palpating.
   b. Use the optimal palpation position.
   c. Passively slacken the target muscle.
   d. Have the client place a hand over their palpating hand.

9. Which of the following bones can be palpated on the anterior side of the wrist, immediately distal to the ulna?
   a. Pisiform
   b. Hamate
   c. Scaphoid
   d. Radius

10. Which of the following structures is the most posterior aspect of the pelvic bone and can be located and palpated approximately 2 inches from the midline of the superior aspect (base) of the sacrum?
    a. Anterior superior iliac spine (ASIS)
    b. Sacroiliac joint
    c. Posterior superior iliac spine (PSIS)
    d. Sacral tubercle

Score: __/10

COLORING & LABELING

Use crayons or felt-tipped markers to color the muscles. Use the word banks to fill in the numbers that correspond to the names of the muscles, bones, and bony landmarks in the blanks provided.

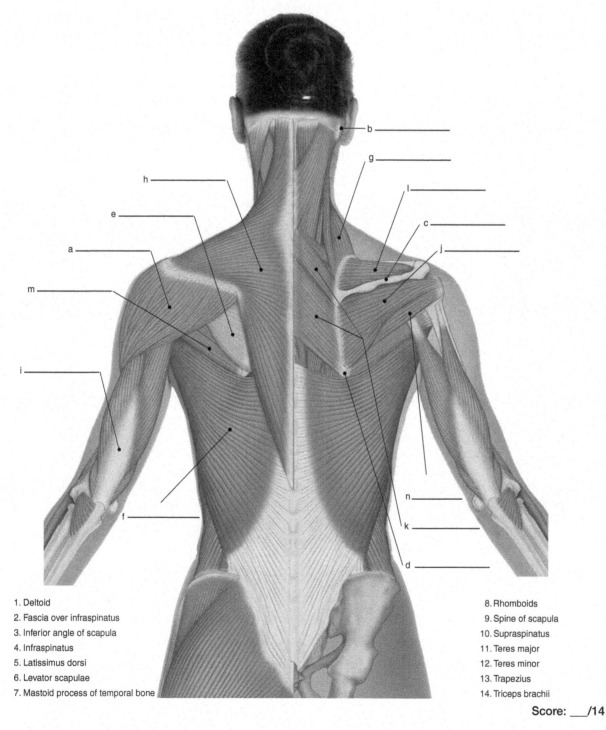

1. Deltoid
2. Fascia over infraspinatus
3. Inferior angle of scapula
4. Infraspinatus
5. Latissimus dorsi
6. Levator scapulae
7. Mastoid process of temporal bone

8. Rhomboids
9. Spine of scapula
10. Supraspinatus
11. Teres major
12. Teres minor
13. Trapezius
14. Triceps brachii

Score: ___/14

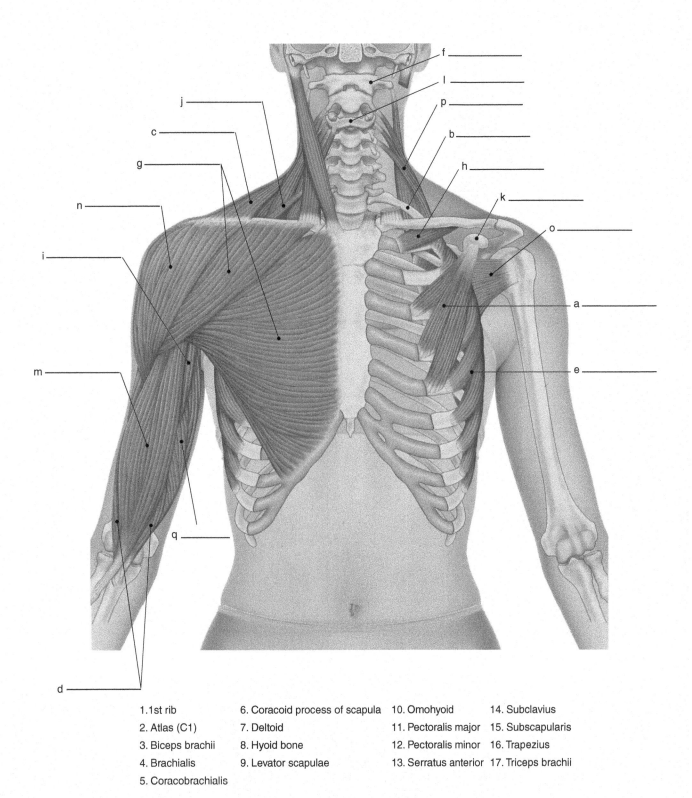

1. 1st rib
2. Atlas (C1)
3. Biceps brachii
4. Brachialis
5. Coracobrachialis

6. Coracoid process of scapula
7. Deltoid
8. Hyoid bone
9. Levator scapulae

10. Omohyoid
11. Pectoralis major
12. Pectoralis minor
13. Serratus anterior

14. Subclavius
15. Subscapularis
16. Trapezius
17. Triceps brachii

Score: ___/17

Chapter **6** **Muscles of the Shoulder Girdle and Arm**

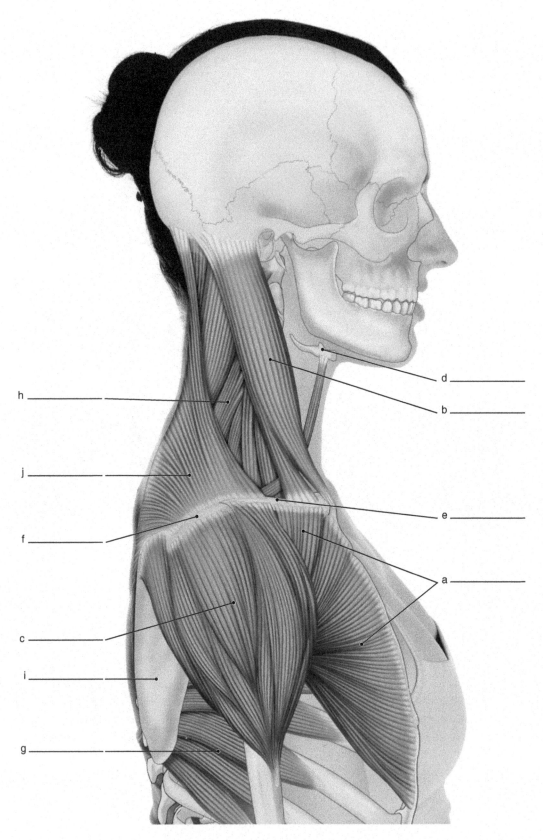

h _____

j _____

f _____

c _____

i _____

g _____

d _____

b _____

e _____

a _____

1. Acromion process of scapula   3. Deltoid   5. Levator scapulae   7. Scapula   9. Sternocleidomastoid

2. Clavicle   4. Hyoid bone   6. Pectoralis major   8. Serratus anterior 10. Trapezius

Score: ___/10

Section 1 tests your knowledge of muscles covered in pages 146-161 of the *Know the Body* textbook.

KNOW YOUR MUSCLES

Fill in the blanks with the name of the muscle(s) shown.

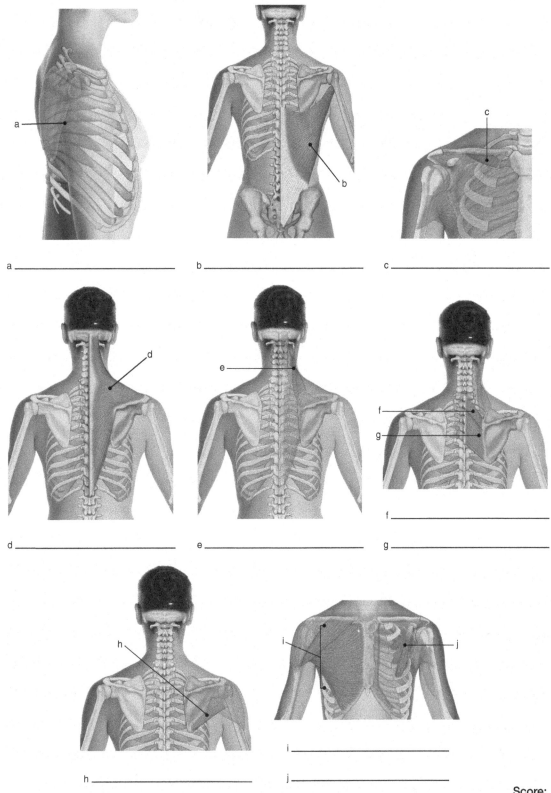

a _____   b _____   c _____

d _____   e _____   f _____

g _____

h _____   i _____

j _____

Score: ___/10

Chapter **6** **Muscles of the Shoulder Girdle and Arm**

Match the muscle name from the right column to its meaning in the left column. Write your answer in the space provided. Each choice can be used only once.

Meaning	**Muscle name**
_____ 1. Trapezoid shape	a. Pectoralis minor
_____ 2. Bigger diamond-shaped muscle	b. Levator scapulae
_____ 3. Smaller diamond-shaped muscle	c. Teres major
_____ 4. Elevates the scapula	d. Rhomboid major
_____ 5. Notched shape and more anterior	e. Pectoralis major
_____ 6. Larger muscle of chest	f. Serratus anterior
_____ 7. Smaller muscle of chest	g. Trapezius
_____ 8. Under the clavicle	h. Latissimus dorsi
_____ 9. Widest muscle of the back	i. Subclavius
_____ 10. Round and large	j. Rhomboid minor

Score: ___/10

MATCHING ATTACHMENTS

Match each muscle from the word bank with its attachments. Write the answer in the column labeled *Muscle*. Each choice can be used only once.

Trapezius	Serratus anterior	Pectoralis major
Rhomboids	Subclavius	Pectoralis minor
Teres major	Levator scapulae	Latissimus dorsi

Attachments	Muscle
1. External occipital protuberance, medial one third of the superior nuchal line of the occiput, nuchal ligament, and spinous processes of C7 – T12 *to the* Lateral one third of the clavicle, acromion process and the spine of the scapula	
2. Spinous processes of C7 – T5 *to the* Medial border of the scapula from the root of the spine of the scapula to the inferior angle of the scapula	
3. Transverse process of C1–C4 *to the* Medial border of the scapula, between the superior angle and the root of the spine of the scapula	

4. Ribs 1 through 9 *to the* Anterior surface of the entire medial border of the scapula	
5. Medial clavicle, sternum, and the costal cartilages of ribs one through seven *to the* Lateral lip of the bicipital groove of the humerus	
6. Ribs 3 through 5 *to the* Coracoid process of the scapula	
7. 1st rib *to the* Clavicle	
8. Inferior angle of the scapula, spinous processes of T7-L5, posterior sacrum, and the posterior iliac crest *to the* Medial lip of the bicipital groove of the humerus	
9. Inferior angle and inferior lateral border of the scapula *to the* Medial lip of the bicipital groove of the humerus	

Score: ___/9

THE BIG PICTURE – FUNCTIONAL GROUPS

Fill in the blanks with 1) the direction of movement, 2) the body part that is moving, and 3) the joint at which movement occurs.

1. If a muscle attaches to the scapula and its other attachment is superior to the scapula, what action can it perform?

   _____ of the _____ at the _____ joint(s).

2. If a muscle attaches to the scapula and its other attachment is inferior to the scapula, what action can it perform?

   _____ of the _____ at the _____ joint(s).

3. If a muscle attaches to the scapula and its other attachment is anterior to the scapula, what action can it perform?

   _____ of the _____ at the _____ joint(s).

4. If a muscle attaches to the scapula and its other attachment is posterior to the scapula, what action can it perform?

   _____ of the _____ at the _____ joint(s).

5. If a muscle crosses the glenohumeral joint anteriorly with a vertical direction to its fibers, what action can it perform?

   _____ of the _____ at the _____ joint(s).

6. If a muscle crosses the glenohumeral joint posteriorly with a vertical direction to its fibers, what action can it perform?

   _____ of the _____ at the _____ joint(s).

7. If a muscle crosses the glenohumeral joint medially (inferiorly, below the center of the joint), what action can it perform?

   _____ of the _____ at the _____ joint(s).

69

8. If a muscle wraps around the humerus from medial to lateral, anterior to the glenohumeral joint, what action can it perform?

_____ of the _____ at the _____ joint(s).

MATCHING ACTIONS

Place the corresponding joint action letter(s) in the blank(s) next to the muscle. Some letters will be used more than once. The number of blanks next to each muscle name indicates the number of letters that should be placed next to that muscle.

Note: The scapula moves at the scapulocostal joint; arm at the glenohumeral joint; clavicle at the sternoclavicular joint; and the first rib at the sternocostal and costospinal joints.

Joint Action

a. Elevates the scapula

b. Depresses the scapula

c. Retracts the scapula

d. Protracts the scapula

e. Rotates the scapula upward

f. Rotates the scapula downward

g. Flexes the arm

h. Extends the arm

i. Abducts the arm

j. Adducts the arm

k. Medially rotates the arm

l. Laterally rotates the arm

m. Depresses the clavicle

n. Elevates the 1st rib

o. Elevates ribs 3 through 5

p. Extends the neck

q. Extends the head and neck

r. Laterally fexes the neck

s. Laterally flexes the head and neck

t. Ipsilaterally rotates the neck

u. Contralaterally rotates the head and neck

Muscle

1. Upper trapezius ___ ___ ___ ___ ___ ___

2. Middle trapezius ___

3. Lower trapezius ___ ___

4. Rhomboids ___ ___ ___

5. Levator scapulae ___ ___ ___ ___ ___

6. Serratus anterior ___ ___

7. Pectoralis major ___ ___ ___ ___ ___

8. Pectoralis minor ___ ___ ___

9. Subclavius ___ ___

10. Latissimus dorsi ___ ___ ___

11. Teres major ___ ___ ___

THE LONG AND THE SHORT OF IT – EXERCISE 1

For each joint action given, indicate whether the muscle shortens or lengthens.

1. Rhomboids: protraction of the scapula: _____

2. Pectoralis major: abduction of the arm: _____

3. Latissimus dorsi: medial rotation of the arm: _____

4. Left levator scapulae: left lateral flexion of the neck: _____

5. Right upper trapezius: left rotation of the neck: _____

Score: ___/5

THE LONG AND THE SHORT OF IT – EXERCISE 2

For each joint action given, fill in the blanks with a muscle that shortens and a muscle that lengthens.

1. Protraction of the scapula:

   Shortens: _____   Lengthens: _____

2. Retraction of the scapula:

   Shortens: _____   Lengthens: _____

3. Elevation of the scapula:

   Shortens: _____   Lengthens: _____

4. Downward rotation of the scapula:

   Shortens: _____   Lengthens: _____

5. Flexion of the arm:

   Shortens: _____   Lengthens: _____

Score: ___/10

MOVERS & ANTAGONISTS – EXERCISE 1

For each joint action stated, fill in the blank with the mover and antagonist of that joint action. Please choose your mover/antagonist pairs from the word bank below. Each pair can be used only once.

   Upper trapezius/Pectoralis minor

   Upper trapezius/Lower trapezius

   Serratus anterior/Rhomboids

   Teres major/Pectoralis major

1. Protraction of the scapula at the scapulocostal joint:

   _____

2. Extension of the arm at the glenohumeral joint:

   _____

Chapter **6** **Muscles of the Shoulder Girdle and Arm**

3. Elevation of the scapula at the scapulocostal joint:

_____

4. Upward rotation of the scapula at the scapulocostal joint:

_____

Score: ___/4

MOVERS & ANTAGONISTS – EXERCISE 2

For each joint action illustrated, the body part is being *slowly* moved in the direction indicated by the arrow. Circle whether the functional muscle group of the pair provided is contracting or relaxed. Then circle *how* the muscle group that is working is contracting (concentrically or eccentrically).

1.
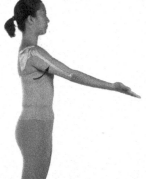

Movement:

Flexion of the arm at the glenohumeral joint

Flexors: contracting/relaxed

Extensors: contracting/relaxed

What type of contraction is occurring
concentric/eccentric

2.
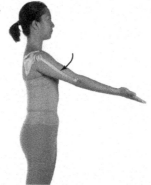

Movement:

Extension of the arm at the glenohumeral joint

Flexors: contracting/relaxed

Extensors: contracting/relaxed

What type of contraction is occurring?
concentric/eccentric

3.
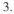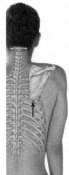

Movement:

Elevation of the scapula at the scapulocostal joint

Elevators: contracting/relaxed

Depressors: contracting/relaxed

What type of contraction is occurring?
concentric/eccentric

4.
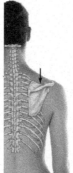

Movement:

Depression of the scapula at the scapulocostal joint

Elevators: contracting/relaxed

Depressors: contracting/relaxed

What type of contraction is occurring?
concentric/eccentric

Score: ___/12

MUSCLE STABILIZATIONS

Circle the letter of the best answer to the question.

1. Which of the following muscles can stabilize the shoulder girdle?
   a. Levator scapulae
   b. Rhomboids
   c. Trapezius
   d. All of the above

2. Which of the following muscles can stabilize the cervical spine?
   a. Serratus anterior
   b. Pectoralis minor
   c. Levator scapulae
   d. Subclavius

3. Which of the following muscles can stabilize the clavicle?
   a. Latissimus dorsi
   b. Levator scapulae
   c. Rhomboids
   d. Subclavius

4. Which of the following muscles can stabilize the glenohumeral joint?
   a. Trapezius
   b. Teres major
   c. Pectoralis minor
   d. All of the above

Score: ___/4

YOU'VE GOT NERVE!

For each muscle listed below, write the name of the corresponding innervation from the word bank provided. Choices can be used more than once.

Spinal accessory nerve (CN XI)

Dorsal scapular nerve

Medial and lateral pectoral nerves

Long thoracic nerve

Thoracodorsal nerve

1. Trapezius _____

2. Rhomboids _____

3. Serratus anterior _____

4. Levator scapulae _____

5. Pectoralis major _____

6. Latissimus dorsi _____

Score: ___/6

Chapter **6** **Muscles of the Shoulder Girdle and Arm**

Fill in the blank with the best answer.

1. Name a muscle for which the palpation protocol is to place the client's hand in the small of the back.

   _____

2. What muscle is palpated by having the client supine and asking them to reach their hand toward the ceiling?

   _____

3. Name a muscle that is superficial and palpable in the posterior triangle of the neck.

   _____

4. What muscle is palpated by curling your palpating finger pads around the clavicle?

   _____

5. What muscle is palpated immediately distal to the coracoid process of the scapula and deep to the pectoralis major?

   _____

6. What muscle is palpated with the client prone, arm abducted to 90 degrees, and scapula retracted?

   _____

Score: ___/6

CLINICALLY SPEAKING

Fill in the blank with the best answer for the treatment consideration question.

1. Carrying a bag on the shoulder, crimping/holding a phone between the ear and shoulder, or holding the arm in abduction would overuse and aggravate what muscle?

   _____

2. Weakness of the rhomboids would most likely result in what postural distortion pattern?

   _____

3. What muscle often becomes tight and visible in the posterior triangle of the neck in middle or older age?

   _____

4. Weakness of what muscle results in "winged scapulae"?

   _____

5. What muscle, if tight, can impinge the brachial plexus of nerves against the rib cage?

   _____

Score: ___/5

Fill in the blank with the best answer to the question.

1. What muscle attaches from the coracoid process of the scapula to ribs 3 through 5?

   _____

2. The rhomboids are deep to what muscle? _____

3. What muscles attach to the medial border of the scapula?

   _____

4. What muscle can elevate and depress the scapula at the scapulocostal joint?

   _____

5. Name two muscles that can upwardly rotate the scapula at the scapulocostal joint.

   _____

6. What is the broad flat muscle that is superficial in the posterior neck and trunk?

   _____

7. What muscles are known as the *Christmas Tree Muscles?* _____

8. What muscle usually blends into the rhomboids? _____

9. What muscle has a twist in its mid belly? _____

10. What muscle has the same humeral actions as the latissimus dorsi? _____

11. What muscle is located within the anterior axillary fold of tissue?

    _____

12. What muscle is located between the clavicle and 1st rib? _____

13. What muscle is known as the *swimmer's muscle?* _____

14. What muscle of the glenohumeral joint attaches into the thoracolumbar fascia?

    _____

Score: ___/14

Use the clues to complete the crossword puzzle.

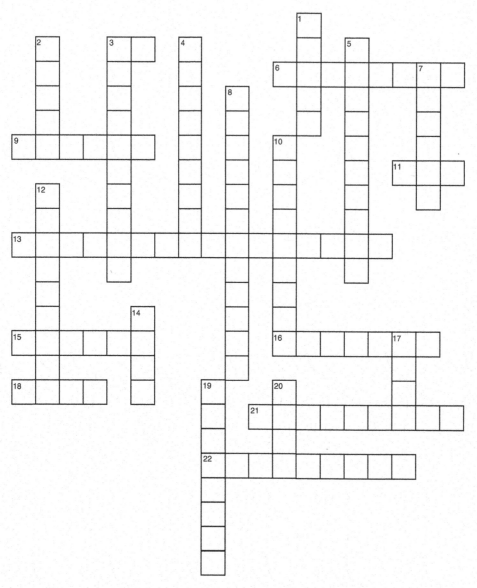

ACROSS

3 Most superior attachment of the rhomboids
6 Serratus anterior attaches to this side of the scapula
9 The pectoralis major and latissimus dorsi border this area
11 "Clavicle" means _____
13 What muscle in the lateral trunk, when well-developed, looks like ribs? (2 words)
15 These trapezial fibers do not rotate the scapula
16 Insertion (distal attachment) of levator scapulae
18 Innervates the trapezius
21 Groove attachment of pectoralis major
22 Sagittal plane glenohumeral joint action of the teres major

DOWN

1 Smaller
2 Larger
3 Head of pectoralis major
4 Located medial to the scapula
5 Attaches to inferior angle of scapula (2 words)
7 Thoracic _____ syndrome
8 The trapezius can be _____ to itself
10 Attaches to the external occipital protuberance
12 Pectoralis minor's action on ribs
14 Location of pectoralis minor to pectoralis major
17 Neck rotation of right upper trapezius
19 Closer to the front
20 The serratus anterior attaches to ribs one through _____

Score: ___/23

Fill in the blank with the best answer for the clinical case study questions.

1. What muscle would likely be tight in a client who has rounded shoulders and is experiencing tingling in the hand?

   _____

2. What two muscles would be most important to assess in a client who is a desk worker who does a lot of phone work and is experiencing a tight neck and headaches?

   _____

3. What three muscles are likely short and tight in a client whose posture shows the clavicle collapsed against the

   ribcage? _____

4. What muscle should be assessed in a client who swims the freestyle stroke every day and is experiencing low back

   pain? _____

Score: ___/4

Section 2 tests your knowledge of muscles covered in pages 162-177 of the *Know the Body* textbook.

KNOW YOUR MUSCLES

Fill in the blank with the name of the muscles shown.

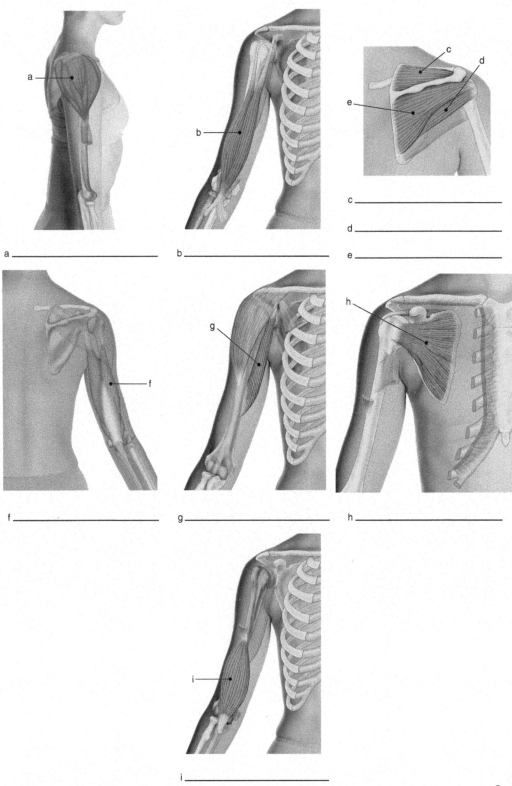

a _____

b _____

c _____

d _____

e _____

f _____

g _____

h _____

i _____

Score: ___/9

WHAT'S IN A NAME?

Match the muscle name from the right column to its meaning in the left column. Write your answer in the space provided. Each choice can be used only once.

Meaning

_____ 1. Attaches to supraspinous fossa of scapula

_____ 2. Attaches to infraspinous fossa of scapula

_____ 3. Round and small

_____ 4. Attaches to subscapular fossa of scapula

_____ 5. Triangular shape

_____ 6. Attaches to coracoid process of scapula and arm

_____ 7. Two-headed muscle overlying arm

_____ 8. Refers to the arm

_____ 9. Three-headed muscle overlying arm

_____ 10. Elbow

Muscle name

a. Deltoid

b. Teres minor

c. Infraspinatus

d. Anconeus

e. Supraspinatus

f. Brachialis

g. Triceps brachii

h. Coracobrachialis

i. Biceps brachii

j. Subscapularis

Score: ___/10

MATCHING ATTACHMENTS

Match each muscle from the word bank with its attachments. Write the answer in the column labeled *Muscle*. Each choice can be used only once.

Deltoid	Infraspinatus	Teres minor
Subscapularis	Supraspinatus	Brachialis
Coracobrachialis	Triceps brachii	Biceps brachii
Anconeus		

Attachments	Muscle
1. Supraspinous fossa of the scapula *to the* Greater tubercle of the humerus	
2. Infraspinous fossa of the scapula *to the* Greater tubercle of the humerus	
3. Superior lateral border of the scapula *to the* Greater tubercle of the humerus	
4. Subscapular fossa of the scapula *to the* Lesser tubercle of the humerus	

Chapter **6** **Muscles of the Shoulder Girdle and Arm**

5. Lateral clavicle, acromion process, and the spine of the scapula *to the* Deltoid tuberosity of the humerus	
6. Coracoid process of the scapula *to the* Medial shaft of the humerus	
7. Long Head: Supraglenoid tubercle of the scapula *and* Short Head: Coracoid process of the scapula *to the* Radial tuberosity	
8. Distal half of the anterior shaft of the humerus *to the* Ulnar tuberosity	
9. Long Head: Infraglenoid tubercle of the scapula *and* Lateral Head: Posterior shaft of the humerus *and* Medial (Deep) Head: Posterior shaft of the humerus *to the* Olecranon process of the ulna	
10. Lateral epicondyle of the humerus *to the* Posterior proximal ulna	

Score: ___/10

THE BIG PICTURE – FUNCTIONAL GROUPS

Fill in the blanks with 1) the direction of movement, 2) the body part that is moving, and 3) the joint at which movement is occurring.

1. If a muscle crosses the glenohumeral joint anteriorly with a vertical direction to its fibers, what action can it perform?

   _____ of the _____ at the _____ joint(s).

2. If a muscle crosses the glenohumeral joint posteriorly with a vertical direction to its fibers, what action can it perform?

   _____ of the _____ at the _____ joint(s).

3. If a muscle crosses the glenohumeral joint medially (inferiorly, below the center of the joint), what action can it perform?

   _____ of the _____ at the _____ joint(s).

4. If a muscle crosses the glenohumeral joint laterally (superiorly, over the center of the joint), what action can it perform?

   _____ of the _____ at the _____ joint(s).

5. If a muscle wraps around the humerus from medial to lateral, posterior to the glenohumeral joint, what action can it perform?

   _____ of the _____ at the _____ joint(s).

6. If a muscle wraps around the humerus from medial to lateral, anterior to the glenohumeral joint, what action can it perform?

_____ of the _____ at the _____ joint(s).

7. If a muscle crosses the elbow joint anteriorly with a vertical direction to its fibers, what action can it perform?

_____ of the _____ at the _____ joint(s).

8. If a muscle crosses the elbow joint posteriorly with a vertical direction to its fibers, what action can it perform?

_____ of the _____ at the _____ joint(s).

9. When the hand (and therefore the forearm) is fixed by holding onto an immovable object, what type of action occurs?

_____.

Score: ___/9

MATCHING ACTIONS

Place the corresponding joint action letter(s) in the blank(s) next to the muscle. The number of blanks next to each muscle name indicates the number of letters that should be placed next to that muscle.
Note: The arm moves at the glenohumeral joint, and the forearm moves at the elbow and/or radioulnar joints.

Joint Action

a. Flexes the arm

b. Extends the arm

c. Abducts the arm

d. Adducts the arm

e. Laterally rotates the arm

f. Medially rotates the arm

g. Horizontally flexes the arm

h. Horizontally extends the arm

i. Rotates the scapula downward

j. Flexes the forearm

k. Extends the forearm

l. Supinates the forearm

Muscle

1. Supraspinatus ____ ____

2. Infraspinatus ____

3. Teres minor ____

4. Subscapularis ____

5. Entire deltoid ____ ____

6. Anterior deltoid ____ ____ ____ ____

7. Posterior deltoid ____ ____ ____ ____

8. Coracobrachialis ____ ____

9. Biceps brachii ____ ____ ____

10. Brachialis ____

11. Triceps brachii ____ ____

12. Anconeus ____

Score: ___/22

Chapter **6** **Muscles of the Shoulder Girdle and Arm**

THE LONG AND THE SHORT OF IT – EXERCISE 1

For each joint action given, indicate whether the muscle shortens or lengthens.

1. Teres minor: lateral rotation of the arm: _____

2. Coracobrachialis: abduction of the arm: _____

3. Biceps brachii: extension of the elbow joint: _____

4. Anterior deltoid: abduction of the glenohumeral joint: _____

5. Subscapularis: lateral rotation of the glenohumeral joint: _____

Score: ___/5

THE LONG AND THE SHORT OF IT – EXERCISE 2

For each joint action given, fill in the blanks with a muscle that shortens and a muscle that lengthens.

1. Flexion of the arm:

   Shortens: _____   Lengthens: _____

2. Extension of the arm:

   Shortens: _____   Lengthens: _____

3. Lateral rotation of the arm:

   Shortens: _____   Lengthens: _____

4. Adduction of the arm:

   Shortens: _____   Lengthens: _____

5. Flexion of the forearm:

   Shortens: _____   Lengthens: _____

Score: ___/10

MOVERS & ANTAGONISTS – EXERCISE 1

For each joint action stated, fill in the blank with a mover and antagonist of that joint action. Please choose mover/antagonist pairs from the word bank below. Each pair can be used once and only once.

   Anterior deltoid/Posterior deltoid

   Infraspinatus/Subscapularis

   Triceps brachii/Brachialis

   Supraspinatus/Coracobrachialis

1. Lateral rotation of the arm at the glenohumeral joint:

   _____

2. Abduction of the arm at the glenohumeral joint:

   _____

3. Extension of the forearm at the elbow joint:

_____

4. Flexion of the arm at the glenohumeral joint:

_____

Score: ___/4

MOVERS & ANTAGONISTS – EXERCISE 2

For each joint action illustrated, the body part is being *slowly* moved in the direction indicated by the arrow. Circle whether the functional muscle group of the pair provided is contracting or relaxed. Then circle *how* the muscle group that is working is contracting (concentrically or eccentrically).

1.

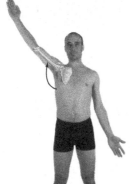

Movement:

Abduction of the arm at the glenohumeral joint

Abductors: contracting/relaxed

Adductors: contracting/relaxed

What type of contraction is occurring?
concentric/eccentric

2.

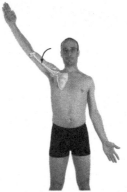

Movement:

Adduction of the arm at the glenohumeral joint

Abductors: contracting/relaxed

Adductors: contracting/relaxed

What type of contraction is occurring?
concentric/eccentric

3.

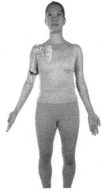

Movement:

Lateral rotation of the arm at the glenohumeral joint

Lateral rotators: contracting/relaxed

Medial rotators: contracting/relaxed

What type of contraction is occurring?
concentric/eccentric

4.

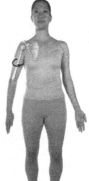

Movement:

Medial rotation of the arm at the glenohumeral joint

Lateral rotators: contracting/relaxed

Medial rotators: contracting/relaxed

What type of contraction is occurring?
concentric/eccentric

Score: ___/12

83

MUSCLE STABILIZATIONS

Circle the letter of the best answer to the question.

1. Which of the following muscles can stabilize the glenohumeral joint?
   a. Supraspinatus
   b. Infraspinatus
   c. Subscapularis
   d. All of the above

2. Which of the following muscles can stabilize the radioulnar joints?
   a. Biceps brachii
   b. Brachialis
   c. Anconeus
   d. Deltoid

3. Which of the following muscles can stabilize both the glenohumeral and elbow joints?
   a. Coracobrachialis
   b. Infraspinatus
   c. Brachialis
   d. Triceps brachii

4. Which of the following muscles can stabilize the elbow joint?
   a. Teres minor
   b. Coracobrachialis
   c. Anconeus
   d. Subscapularis

Score: ___/4

YOU'VE GOT NERVE!

Write in the name of the corresponding innervation from the word bank provided. Choices can be used more than once.

Axillary nerve

Musculocutaneous nerve

Radial nerve

Suprascapular nerve

Upper and lower subscapular nerves

1. Deltoid _____

2. Infraspinatus _____

3. Biceps brachii _____

4. Triceps brachii _____

5. Brachialis _____

6. Subscapularis _____

Score: ___/6

ARE YOU FEELING IT? – PALPATION

Fill in the blank with the best answer to the palpation question.

1. When engaging and palpating the deltoid, where do you place your resistance hand? _____

2. The distal tendon of the supraspinatus is palpated deep to what muscle? _____

3. What muscles can be palpated along the lateral border of the scapula?

   _____

4. What muscle is palpated on the anterior surface of the scapula and is engaged by asking the client to medially rotate the arm at the glenohumeral joint? _____

5. Which fibers of the deltoid are best engaged and palpated with horizontal flexion of the arm at the glenohumeral joint?

   _____

6. In what position should the forearm at the radioulnar joints be when palpating the brachialis?

   _____

Score: ___/6

CLINICALLY SPEAKING

Fill in the blank with the best answer for the treatment consideration question.

1. The distal tendon of what muscle is commonly injured between the greater tubercle of the humerus and the acromion process of the scapula? _____

2. What muscle(s) is commonly overused and injured by working at a keyboard with the arms isometrically held in abduction and/or flexion? _____

3. What neurovascular structures are located close to the coracobrachialis?

   _____

4. Which head/tendon of the biceps brachii is more often irritated and injured?

   _____

5. The radial nerve can be pinched and injured between the heads of what muscle?

   _____

Score: ___/5

Chapter **6** **Muscles of the Shoulder Girdle and Arm**

Fill in the blank with the best answer to the question.

1. What are the names of the three parts of the deltoid?

   _____

2. From an anterior perspective, what muscle is deep to the biceps brachii in the distal arm?

   _____

3. What is the best way to expose the coracobrachialis for palpation?

   _____

4. Does the biceps brachii attach to the humerus? _____

5. Which two rotator cuff muscles can laterally rotate the arm at the glenohumeral joint?

   _____

6. This rotator cuff muscle is located immediately superior to the teres major at the lateral border of the scapula.

   _____

7. Much of the infraspinatus is deep to what muscle? _____

8. The belly of the supraspinatus is deep to what muscle? _____

9. True or false: The brachialis pronates the forearm. _____

10. True or false: Both heads of the biceps brachii cross the glenohumeral joint. _____

11. What nerve innervates the majority of the muscles of the anterior arm? _____

12. Name two muscles that attach to the coracoid process of the scapula. _____

13. What muscle is engaged and palpated when the client is seated and pressing their forearm down against their thigh?

    _____

14. What two rotator cuff muscles are palpated with the client prone, the arm resting on the table, and the forearm hanging off the table between the therapist's knees? _____

15. What muscle can be its own antagonist at the glenohumeral joint? _____

Score: ___/15

Use the clues to complete the crossword puzzle.

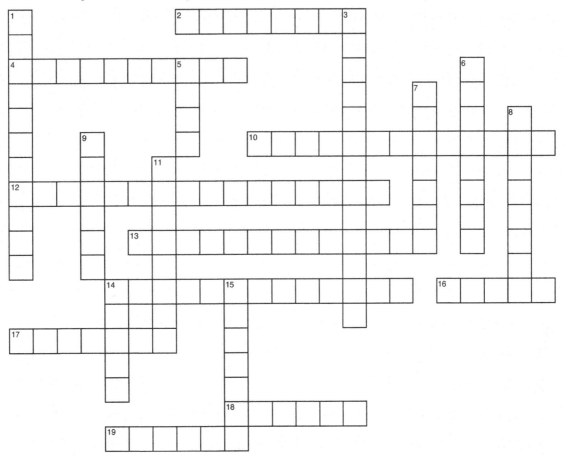

ACROSS

2 Its name means "elbow"
4 Flexes the elbow joint and attaches to the ulnar tuberosity
10 This muscle abducts and flexes the arm
12 The coracobrachialis is pierced by this nerve
13 Located in the infraspinous fossa
14 The most important function of the rotator cuff group
16 Number of rotator cuff muscles that attach to the greater tubercle
17 Its proximal attachments are the same as the trapezius' distal attachments
18 The coracobrachialis can be palpated in this area
19 Innervates the majority of the muscles of the posterior arm and forearm

DOWN

1 This bursa is located next to the supraspinatus
3 The serratus anterior and this muscle are located between the scapula and rib cage
5 The only triceps brachii head that crosses the glenohumeral joint
6 The name deltoid literally means that it resembles the shape of a_____
7 The anconeus assists this muscle
8 All rotator cuff muscles attach to this type of humeral landmark
9 The brachialis is deep to this muscle and helps it looks larger
11 The deltoid's rotation of the scapula at the glenohumeral joint
14 This head of a well-known muscle blends with the coracobrachialis
15 The brachialis is superficial and easily palpable in this region of the arm

Score: ___/19

MINI CASE STUDIES

Fill in the blank with the best answer for the clinical case study questions.

1. What muscle would most likely be injured if a client experiences anterior arm pain when performing "biceps curls" with the forearm in full pronation? _____

2. What two muscles should be assessed if a client presents with shoulder pain and states that he has been doing arm raises to the side with weights?

_____

3. What rotator cuff muscle is most likely shortened adaptively and tightened in a person with rounded shoulders (medially rotated arms)? _____

4. What muscle should be assessed if a client is experiencing pain in the lateral arm, approximately one third of the way down the shaft? _____

Score: ___/4

MNEMONICS

Create your own mnemonic for the muscle group.

Rotator Cuff Group:

Supraspinatus, Infraspinatus, Teres Minor, Subscapularis

Soup In The Miner's Shaft.

Now make one of your own:

S _____ I _____ T _____ M _____ S _____.

Actions of the biceps brachii:

Flexion, Supination, Flexion

Felix Scrubs Faucets.

Now make one of your own:

F _____ S _____ F _____

Major flexors of the elbow joint.

Brachialis, Biceps brachii, Brachioradialis (Note: Brachioradialis is covered in Chapter 7)

Three B's Bend the elBow.

Now make one of your own:

B _____ B _____ B _____

7 Muscles of the Forearm and Hand

COLORING & LABELING

Use crayons or felt-tipped markers to color the muscles. Use the word banks to fill in the numbers that correspond to the names of the muscles, bones, and bony landmarks in the blanks provided.

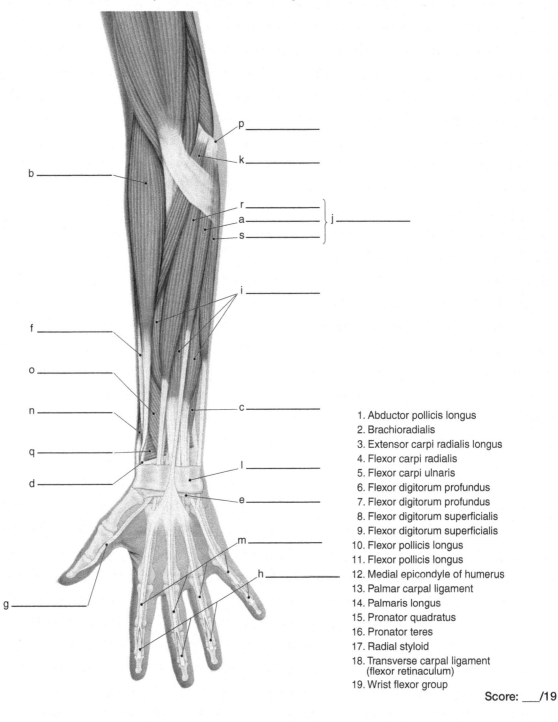

1. Abductor pollicis longus
2. Brachioradialis
3. Extensor carpi radialis longus
4. Flexor carpi radialis
5. Flexor carpi ulnaris
6. Flexor digitorum profundus
7. Flexor digitorum profundus
8. Flexor digitorum superficialis
9. Flexor digitorum superficialis
10. Flexor pollicis longus
11. Flexor pollicis longus
12. Medial epicondyle of humerus
13. Palmar carpal ligament
14. Palmaris longus
15. Pronator quadratus
16. Pronator teres
17. Radial styloid
18. Transverse carpal ligament (flexor retinaculum)
19. Wrist flexor group

Score: ___/19

89

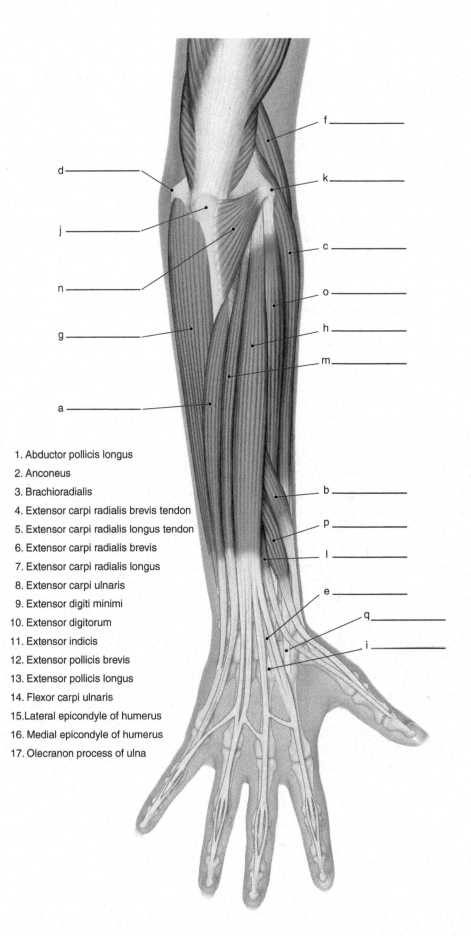

f _____

d _____

k _____

j _____

c _____

n _____

o _____

g _____

h _____

m _____

a _____

1. Abductor pollicis longus
2. Anconeus
3. Brachioradialis
4. Extensor carpi radialis brevis tendon
5. Extensor carpi radialis longus tendon
6. Extensor carpi radialis brevis
7. Extensor carpi radialis longus
8. Extensor carpi ulnaris
9. Extensor digiti minimi
10. Extensor digitorum
11. Extensor indicis
12. Extensor pollicis brevis
13. Extensor pollicis longus
14. Flexor carpi ulnaris
15. Lateral epicondyle of humerus
16. Medial epicondyle of humerus
17. Olecranon process of ulna

b _____

p _____

l _____

e _____

q _____

i _____

Score: ___/17

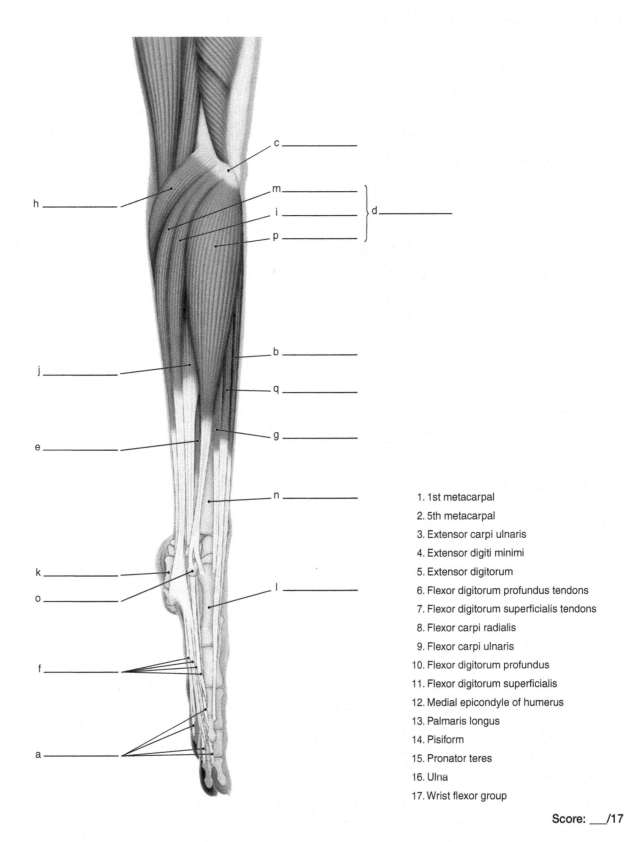

1. 1st metacarpal
2. 5th metacarpal
3. Extensor carpi ulnaris
4. Extensor digiti minimi
5. Extensor digitorum
6. Flexor digitorum profundus tendons
7. Flexor digitorum superficialis tendons
8. Flexor carpi radialis
9. Flexor carpi ulnaris
10. Flexor digitorum profundus
11. Flexor digitorum superficialis
12. Medial epicondyle of humerus
13. Palmaris longus
14. Pisiform
15. Pronator teres
16. Ulna
17. Wrist flexor group

Score: ___/17

Chapter **7   Muscles of the Forearm and Hand**

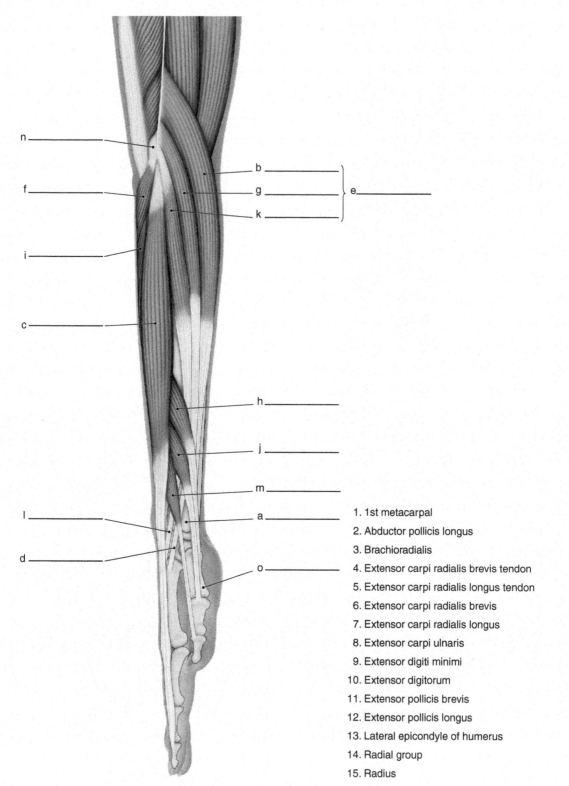

1. 1st metacarpal
2. Abductor pollicis longus
3. Brachioradialis
4. Extensor carpi radialis brevis tendon
5. Extensor carpi radialis longus tendon
6. Extensor carpi radialis brevis
7. Extensor carpi radialis longus
8. Extensor carpi ulnaris
9. Extensor digiti minimi
10. Extensor digitorum
11. Extensor pollicis brevis
12. Extensor pollicis longus
13. Lateral epicondyle of humerus
14. Radial group
15. Radius

Score: ___/15

Chapter **7** **Muscles of the Forearm and Hand**

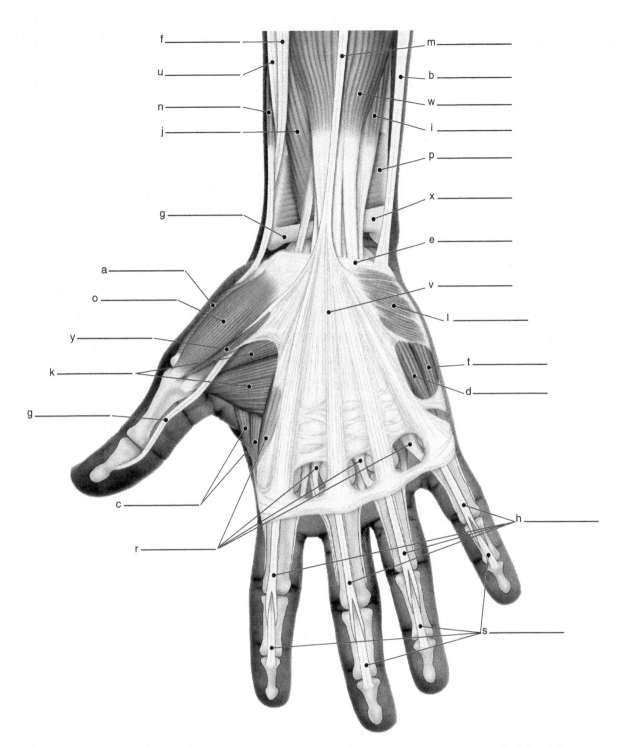

f_____   m_____

u_____   b_____

n_____   w_____
j_____   i_____

                    p_____

g_____   x_____

a_____   e_____

o_____   v_____
                    l_____
y_____
k_____   t_____
                    d_____
g_____

c_____   h_____

r_____   s_____

1. 1st dorsal
   interosseus

2. Abductor pollicis
   longus

3. Abductor
   digiti minimi
   manus

4. Abductor pollicis
   brevis

5. Adductor pollicis

6. Brachioradialis

7. Extensor carpi radialis
   longus

8. Flexor carpi ulnaris

9. Flexor digiti minimi
   manus

10. Flexor digitorum
    profundus

11. Flexor digitorum profundus

12. Flexor digitorum superficialis

13. Flexor digitorum superficialis

14. Flexor pollicis brevis

15. Flexor pollicis longus

16. Flexor pollicis longus

17. Lumbricals manus

18. Opponens pollicis

19. Palmar aponeurosis

20. Palmaris brevis

21. Palmaris longus

22. Pronator quadratus

23. Radius

24. Transverse carpal ligament
    (flexor retinaculum)

25. Ulna

Score: ___/25

93

Section 1 tests your knowledge of muscles covered in pages 198-209 of the *Know the Body* textbook.

KNOW YOUR MUSCLES

Fill in the blank with the name of the muscles shown.

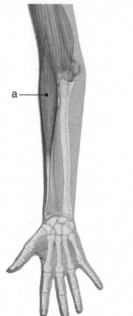

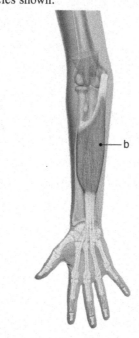

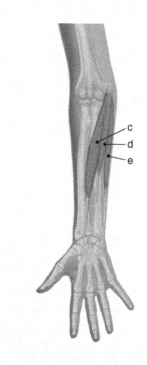

a _____

b _____

c _____

d _____

e _____

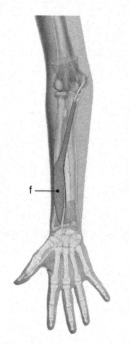

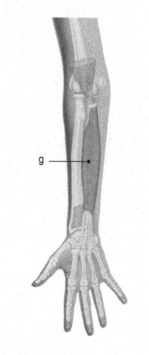

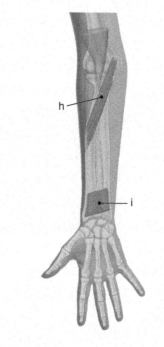

f _____

g _____

h _____

i _____

Chapter **7** **Muscles of the Forearm and Hand**

Score: ___/9

Match the muscle name from the right column to its meaning in the left column. Write your answer in the space provided. Each choice can be used only once.

Meaning

_____ 1. Flexes and ulnar deviates the wrist joint

_____ 2. Square muscle that pronates

_____ 3. Longer flexor of thumb

_____ 4. Flexes and radially deviates the wrist joint

_____ 5. More superficial flexor of fingers

_____ 6. Attaches to the arm and radius

_____ 7. Round muscle that pronates

_____ 8. Deeper flexor of fingers

_____ 9. Longer muscle of the palm

Muscle name

a. Flexor digitorum superficialis

b. Brachioradialis

c. Flexor pollicis longus

d. Flexor carpi radialis

e. Flexor digitorum profundus

f. Pronator teres

g. Pronator quadratus

h. Flexor carpi ulnaris

i. Palmaris longus

Score: ___/9

MATCHING ATTACHMENTS

Match each muscle from the word bank with its attachments. Write the answer in the column labeled *Muscle*. Each choice will be used only once.

Flexor digitorum superficialis   Flexor carpi radialis

Flexor pollicis longus   Pronator quadratus

Flexor carpi ulnaris   Brachioradialis

Flexor digitorum profundus   Palmaris longus

Pronator teres

Attachments	Muscle
1. Medial epicondyle of the humerus via the common flexor tendon *to the* Anterior hand on the radial side	
2. Medial epicondyle of the humerus via the common flexor tendon *to the* Palm of the hand	
3. Medial epicondyle of the humerus via the common flexor tendon, and the ulna *to the* Anterior hand on the ulnar side	
4. Humeral Head: Medial epicondyle of the humerus via the common flexor tendon *and* Ulnar Head: Coronoid process of the ulna *to the* Lateral radius	

95

5. Anterior distal ulna *to the* Anterior distal radius	
6. Lateral supracondylar ridge of the humerus *to the* Styloid process of the radius	
7. Medial epicondyle of the humerus via the common flexor tendon, and the anterior ulna and radius *to the* anterior surfaces of fingers 2 through 5	
8. Medial and anterior ulna *to the* Anterior surfaces of fingers 2 through 5	
9. Anterior surface of the radius and ulna and the medial epicondyle of the humerus *to the* Thumb	

Score: ___/9

THE BIG PICTURE – FUNCTIONAL GROUPS

Fill in the blanks with 1) the direction of movement, 2) the body part that is moving, and 3) the joint at which movement is occurring.

1. If a muscle crosses the wrist joint anteriorly with a vertical direction to its fibers, what action can it perform?

   _____ of the _____ at the _____ joint(s).

2. If a muscle crosses the wrist joint posteriorly with a vertical direction to its fibers, what action can it perform?

   _____ of the _____ at the _____ joint(s).

3. If a muscle crosses the wrist joint radially (on the lateral side) with a vertical direction to its fibers, what action can it perform?

   _____ of the _____ at the _____ joint(s).

4. If a muscle crosses the wrist joint on the ulnar side (medially) with a vertical direction to its fibers, what action can it perform?

   _____ of the _____ at the _____ joint(s).

5. If a muscle crosses the joints of fingers 2 through 5 anteriorly with a vertical direction to its fibers, what action can it perform?

   _____ of the _____ at the _____ joint(s).

6. If a muscle crosses the joints of fingers 2 through 5 posteriorly with a vertical direction to its fibers, what action can it perform?

   _____ of the _____ at the _____ joint(s).

7. If a muscle crosses the radioulnar joints anteriorly with a horizontal orientation to its fibers, what action can it perform?

_____ of the _____ at the _____ joint(s).

8. If a muscle crosses the radioulnar joints posteriorly with a horizontal orientation to its fibers, what action can it perform?

_____ of the _____ at the _____ joint(s).

9. If a muscle crosses the elbow joint anteriorly with a vertical direction to its fibers, what action can it perform?

_____ of the _____ at the _____ joint(s).

10. If a muscle crosses the elbow joint posteriorly with a vertical direction to its fibers, what action can it perform?

_____ of the _____ at the _____ joint(s).

11. If the hand is holding on to an immovable object, and muscles that cross the elbow, radioulnar, wrist, or finger joints contract, what type of actions occur?

_____

Score: ___/11

MATCHING ACTIONS

Place the corresponding joint action letter(s) in the blank(s) next to the muscle. The number of blanks next to each muscle name indicates the number of letters that should be placed next to that muscle.

Note: The forearm moves at the elbow and/or radioulnar joints; the hand at the wrist joint; fingers 2 through 5 at the metacarpophalangeal, proximal interphalangeal, and distal interphalangeal joints; and the thumb at the saddle, metacarpophalangeal and interphalangeal joints.

Joint Action

a. Flexes the forearm

b. Pronates the forearm

c. Supinates the forearm

d. Flexes the hand

e. Radially deviates the hand

f. Ulnarly deviates the hand

g. Flexes the fingers

h. Flexes the thumb

Muscle

1. Flexor carpi radialis ____ ____

2. Palmaris longus ____

3. Flexor carpi ulnaris ____ ____

4. Pronator teres ____ ____

5. Pronator quadratus ____

6. Brachioradialis ____ ____ ____

7. Flexor digitorum superficialis ____ ____

8. Flexor digitorum profundus ____ ____

9. Flexor pollicis longus ____ ____

Score: ___/17

Chapter **7** **Muscles of the Forearm and Hand**

THE LONG AND THE SHORT OF IT – EXERCISE 1

For each joint action given, indicate whether the muscle shortens or lengthens.

1. Flexor carpi radialis: radial deviation of the hand: _____

2. Flexor carpi ulnaris: extension of the wrist joint: _____

3. Pronator teres: extension of the elbow joint: _____

4. Flexor digitorum superficialis: extension of fingers 2 through 5: _____

5. Flexor pollicis longus: flexion of the thumb: _____

Score: ___/5

THE LONG AND THE SHORT OF IT – EXERCISE 2

For each joint action given, fill in the blanks with a muscle that shortens and a muscle that lengthens. Please note that possible answers may be covered in another section or chapter.

1. Flexion of the wrist joint:

   Shortens: _____   Lengthens: _____

2. Extension of the wrist joint:

   Shortens: _____   Lengthens: _____

3. Radial deviation of the hand:

   Shortens: _____   Lengthens: _____

4. Flexion of fingers two through five:

   Shortens: _____   Lengthens: _____

5. Pronation of the forearm:

   Shortens: _____   Lengthens: _____

Score: ___/10

MOVERS & ANTAGONISTS – EXERCISE 1

For each joint action stated, fill in the blank for a mover and antagonist of that joint action. Please choose your mover/antagonist pairs from the word bank below. Each pair can be used once and only once.

Pronator teres/Brachioradialis

Flexor carpi radialis/Flexor carpi ulnaris

1. Radial deviation of the hand at the wrist joint:

   _____

2. Pronation of the forearm at the radioulnar joints:

   _____

Score: ___/2

For each joint action illustrated, the body part is being *slowly* moved in the direction indicated by the arrow. Circle whether the functional muscle group of the pair provided is contracting or relaxed. Then circle *how* the muscle group that is working is contracting (concentrically or eccentrically).

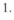

1.

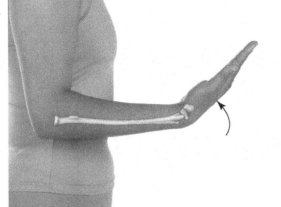

Movement:

Flexion of the hand at the wrist joint

Flexors: contracting/relaxed

Extensors: contracting/relaxed

What type of contraction is occurring?
concentric/eccentric

2.

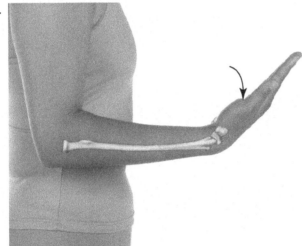

Movement:

Extension of the hand at the wrist joint

Flexors: contracting/relaxed

Extensors: contracting/relaxed

What type of contraction is occurring?
concentric/eccentric

3.

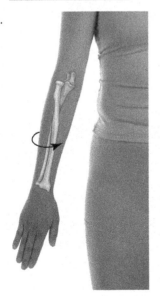

Movement:

Pronation of the forearm at the radioulnar joints

Pronators: contracting/relaxed

Supinators: contracting/relaxed

What type of contraction is occurring?
concentric/eccentric

Score: ___/9

MUSCLE STABILIZATIONS

Circle the letter of the best answer to the question.

1. Which of the following muscles can stabilize the wrist joint?
   a. Brachioradialis
   b. Pronator teres
   c. Palmaris longus
   d. All of the above

2. Which of the following muscles can stabilize the elbow joint?
   a. Pronator teres
   b. Brachioradialis
   c. Flexor digitorum superficialis
   d. All of the above

3. Which of the following muscles can stabilize the radioulnar joints?
   a. Pronator teres
   b. Flexor digitorum profundus
   c. Flexor pollicis longus
   d. Palmaris longus

4. Which of the following muscles can stabilize the saddle joint of the thumb?
   a. Flexor digitorum superficialis
   b. Flexor pollicis longus
   c. Brachioradialis
   d. Flexor digitorum profundus

Score: ___/4

YOU'VE GOT NERVE!

Write in the name of the corresponding innervation from the list provided. Choices will used more than once.

Median nerve

Ulnar nerve

Radial nerve

1. Flexor carpi radialis _____

2. Brachioradialis _____

3. Flexor carpi ulnaris _____

4. Pronator teres _____

5. Flexor digitorum superficialis _____

6. Flexor pollicis longus _____

Score: ___/6

ARE YOU FEELING IT? – PALPATION

Fill in the blank with the best answer to the palpation question.

1. Where is resistance applied when palpating the pronator teres?

_____

2. What two muscles are palpated with the forearm halfway between full pronation and full supination?

_____

3. What joint action engages all three wrist flexors?

_____

4. To engage and palpate the flexor pollicis longus, at which joint do we ask the client to flex the thumb?

_____

5. What finger flexor muscle is palpated directly against the ulna?

_____

Score: ___/5

CLINICALLY SPEAKING

Fill in the blank with the best answer for the treatment consideration question.

1. Overuse of the wrist flexor group would likely cause what condition?

_____

2. What nerve can be entrapped between the two heads of the pronator teres?

_____

3. What are the three Bs of elbow joint flexion?

_____

4. Texting on a cell phone will most likely aggravate and tighten what muscle?

_____

5. The tendons of what muscles travel through the carpal tunnel?

_____

Score: ___/5

MUSCLE MASH-UP

Fill in the blank with the best answer to the question.

1. What are the three muscles of the wrist flexor group?

_____

2. Where does the common flexor tendon attach?

_____

3. Where does the common extensor tendon attach?

_____

4. What muscle is in the intermediate flexor compartment of the forearm?

_____

5. What muscle is directly medial to the pronator teres? _____

6. What is the only muscle that can move the thumb at the interphalangeal joint?

_____

7. What muscle can both pronate and supinate the forearm? _____

8. What is the technical name for tennis elbow?

_____

9. What muscle flexes and performs radial deviation of the hand?

_____

10. Compression due to what muscle can cause cubital tunnel syndrome?

_____

11. What nerve is impinged in carpal tunnel syndrome? _____

12. What are the two long flexors of fingers two through five?

_____

13. What is the common origin (proximal attachment) of the wrist flexor group?

_____

14. Which two muscles attach into the lateral supracondylar ridge of the humerus?

_____

15. What radial group muscle is directly adjacent to the extensor digitorum?

_____

Score: ___/15

CROSSWORD PUZZLE

Use the clues to complete the crossword puzzle.

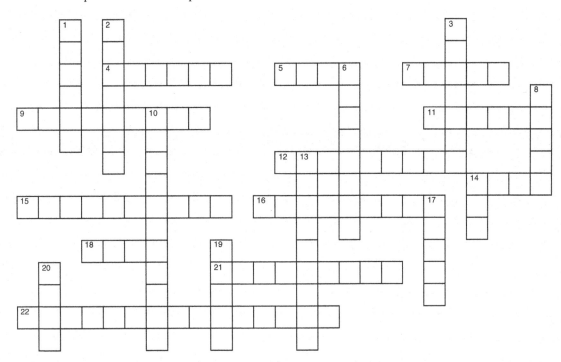

ACROSS

4 Pronator teres can entrap this nerve
5 Profundus
7 Round
9 Square
11 Nerve that innervates the muscles of the posterior forearm
12 Fingers 2-5
14 _____ muscles attach into the common extensor tendon
15 Brachioradialis is sometimes called the _____ muscle
16 Flexors digitorum superficialis and profundus and flexor pollicis longus
18 _____ muscles attach into the common flexor tendon
21 Wrist joint motion that stretches all three wrist flexor muscles
22 Distal attachment is on radial styloid

DOWN

1 "Wad of three" group
2 This head of the flexor pollicis longus is often missing
3 When engaging and palpating the brachioradialis, it is important to place your resistance against the client's distal _____
6 Thumb
8 Deep head of pronator teres
10 Overuse of the muscles of the common extensor tendon (two words)
13 Muscles entirely located within the hand
14 Extrinsic finger flexor that does not cross the elbow joint (acronym)
17 Of the wrist
19 Pronator teres: two _____
20 Radial group muscle next to the brachioradialis (acronym)

Score: ___/22

MINI CASE STUDIES

Fill in the blank with the best answer for the clinical case study questions.

1. A client has been referred to you for therapy of golfer's elbow. Where on the client should you work?

_____

2. What muscles are most important to assess and possibly work in a client who has carpal tunnel syndrome?

_____

Chapter **7** **Muscles of the Forearm and Hand**

3. A client experiences tingling in the hand, but the physician told him that his cervical MRI was negative for nerve impingement. What forearm muscle is most important to assess?

_____

4. What forearm muscle should be assessed in a client who has thumb pain and uses her cell phone a lot?

_____

Score: ___/4

SECTION 2: MUSCLES

KNOW YOUR MUSCLES

Section 2 tests your knowledge of muscle covered in pages 210-220 of the *Know the Body* textbook. Fill in the blank with the name of the muscles shown.

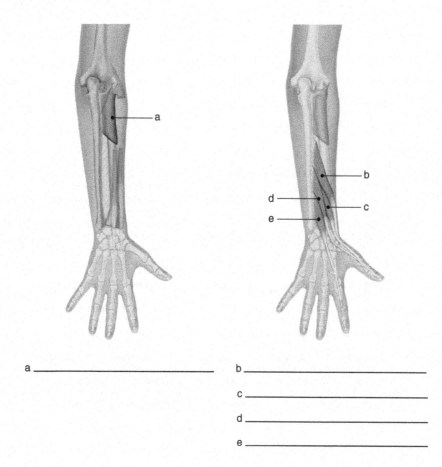

a _____   b _____

c _____

d _____

e _____

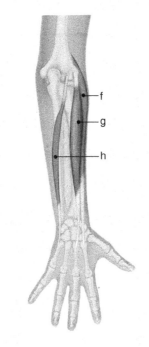
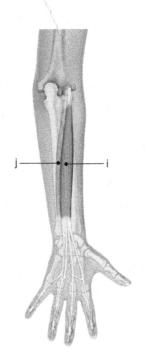

f _____   i _____

g _____   j _____

h _____

Score: ___/10

WHAT'S IN A NAME?

Match the muscle name from the right column to its meaning in the left column. Write your answer in the space provided. Each choice can be used only once.

Meaning

_____ 1. Longer muscle that extends the thumb

_____ 2. Shorter muscle that extends the thumb

_____ 3. Extends and ulnar deviates the wrist joint

_____ 4. Extends digits (fingers 2 through 5)

_____ 5. Longer muscle that extends and radially deviates the wrist joint

_____ 6. Extends the index finger

_____ 7. Longer muscle that abducts the thumb

_____ 8. Supinates

_____ 9. Extends the little digit (finger)

_____ 10. Shorter muscle that extends and radially deviates the wrist joint

Muscle name

a. Abductor pollicis longus

b. Extensor pollicis longus

c. Extensor digitorum

d. Extensor digiti minimi

e. Extensor carpi radialis brevis

f. Extensor indicis

g. Extensor carpi radialis longus

h. Extensor carpi ulnaris

i. Extensor pollicis brevis

j. Supinator

Score: ___/10

Chapter **7** **Muscles of the Forearm and Hand**

Match each muscle from the word bank with its attachments. Write the answer in the column labeled *Muscle*. Each choice will be used only once.

Extensor carpi radialis longus   Extensor digiti minimi

Extensor carpi radialis brevis   Supinator

Extensor pollicis longus   Abductor pollicis longus

Extensor indicis   Extensor carpi ulnaris

Extensor pollicis brevis   Extensor digitorum

Attachments	Muscle
1. Lateral supracondylar ridge of the humerus *to the* Posterior hand on the radial side	
2. Lateral epicondyle of the humerus via the common extensor tendon *to the* Posterior hand on the radial side	
3. Lateral epicondyle of the humerus via the common extensor tendon, and the ulna *to the* Posterior hand on the ulnar side	
4. Lateral epicondyle of the humerus via the common extensor tendon *to the* Phalanges of fingers 2 through 5	
5. Lateral epicondyle of the humerus via the common extensor tendon *to the* Phalanges of the little finger (finger 5)	
6. Lateral epicondyle of the humerus and the proximal ulna *to the* Proximal radius	
7. Posterior radius and ulna *to the* Thumb	
8. Posterior radius *to the* Thumb	
9. Posterior ulna *to the* Thumb	
10. Posterior ulna *to the* Index finger (finger 2)	

Score: ___/10

THE BIG PICTURE – FUNCTIONAL GROUPS

Fill in the blanks with 1) the direction of movement, 2) the body part that is moving, and 3) the joint at which movement is occurring.

1. If a muscle crosses the wrist joint anteriorly with a vertical direction to its fibers, what action can it perform?

   _____ of the _____ at the _____ joint(s).

2. If a muscle crosses the wrist joint posteriorly with a vertical direction to its fibers, what action can it perform?

   _____ of the _____ at the _____ joint(s).

3. If a muscle crosses the wrist joint radially (on the lateral side) with a vertical direction to its fibers, what action can it perform?

   _____ of the _____ at the _____ joint(s).

4. If a muscle crosses the wrist joint on the ulnar side (medially) with a vertical direction to its fibers, what action can it perform?

   _____ of the _____ at the _____ joint(s).

5. If a muscle crosses the metacarpophalangeal joints of fingers two through five posteriorly with a vertical direction to its fibers, what action can it perform?

   _____ of the _____ at the _____ joint(s).

6. If a muscle crosses the radioulnar joints posteriorly with a horizontal orientation to its fibers, what action can it perform?

   _____ of the _____ at the _____ joint(s).

7. If a muscle crosses the carpometacarpal joint of the thumb on the anterior side, what action can it perform?

   _____ of the _____ at the _____ joint(s).

8. If a muscle crosses the carpometacarpal joint of the thumb on the lateral side, what action can it perform?

   _____ of the _____ at the _____ joint(s).

Score: ___/8

MATCHING ACTIONS

Place the corresponding joint action letter(s) in the blank(s) next to the muscle. The number of blanks next to each muscle name indicates the number of letters that should be placed next to that muscle.

Note: The forearm moves at the elbow and/or radioulnar joints; the hand at the wrist joint; fingers 2 through 5 at the metacarpophalangeal, proximal interphalangeal, and distal interphalangeal joints; and the thumb at the saddle, metacarpophalangeal and interphalangeal joints.

Joint Action

a. Supinates the forearm

b. Extends the hand

c. Radially deviates the hand

Muscle

1. Extensor carpi radialis longus ____ ____

2. Extensor carpi radialis brevis ____ ____

3. Extensor carpi ulnaris ____ ____

107

d. Ulnarly deviates the hand

e. Extends the fingers

f. Extends the thumb

g. Abducts the thumb

4. Extensor digitorum ___ ___

5. Extensor digiti minimi ___ ___

6. Supinator ___

7. Abductor pollicis longus ___ ___

8. Extensor pollicis brevis ___ ___

9. Extensor pollicis longus ___

10. Extensor indicis ___

Score: ___/17

THE LONG AND THE SHORT OF IT – EXERCISE 1

For each joint action given, indicate whether the muscle shortens or lengthens.

1. Extensor carpi radialis longus: flexion of the hand: _____

2. Extensor carpi ulnaris: ulnar deviation of the hand: _____

3. Extensor digitorum: flexion of fingers two through five: _____

4. Supinator: pronation of the forearm: _____

5. Abductor pollicis longus: abduction of the thumb: _____

Score: ___/5

THE LONG AND THE SHORT OF IT – EXERCISE 2

For each joint action given, fill in the blanks with a muscle that shortens and a muscle that lengthens. Please note that possible answers may be covered in another section or chapter.

1. Flexion of the wrist joint:

   Shortens: _____   Lengthens: _____

2. Extension of the wrist joint:

   Shortens: _____   Lengthens: _____

3. Radial deviation of the hand:

   Shortens: _____   Lengthens: _____

4. Ulnar deviation of the hand:

   Shortens: _____   Lengthens: _____

5. Pronation of the forearm:

   Shortens: _____   Lengthens: _____

Score: ___/10

For each joint action stated, fill in the blank for a mover and antagonist of that joint action. Please choose your mover/ antagonist pairs from the word bank below. Each pair can be used only once.

Flexor pollicis longus/Extensor pollicis brevis '

Extensor carpi radialis brevis/Flexor carpi ulnaris

Extensor carpi ulnaris/Extensor carpi radialis longus

Extensor digitorum/Flexor digitorum superficialis

Supinator/Pronator quadratus

1. Extension of the hand at the wrist joint:

_____

2. Supination of the forearm at the radioulnar joints:

_____

3. Ulnar deviation of the hand at the wrist joint:

_____

4. Radial deviation of the hand at the wrist joint:

_____

5. Flexion of the thumb at the carpometacarpal joint:

_____

Score: ___/5

For each joint action illustrated, the body part is being *slowly* moved in the direction indicated by the arrow. Circle whether the functional muscle group of the pair provided is contracting or relaxed. Then circle *how* the muscle group that is working is contracting (concentrically or eccentrically).

1.

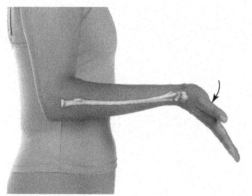

Movement:

Extension of the hand at the wrist joint

    Extensors: contracting/relaxed

    Flexors: contracting/relaxed

    What type of contraction is occurring?
    concentric/eccentric

2.

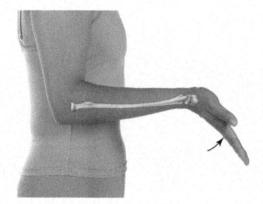

Movement:

Flexion of the hand at the wrist joint

    Flexors: contracting/relaxed

    Extensors: contracting/relaxed

    What type of contraction is occurring?
    concentric/eccentric

3.

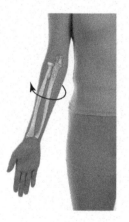

Movement:

Supination of the forearm at the radioulnar joints

    Pronators: contracting/relaxed

    Supinators: contracting/relaxed

    What type of contraction is occurring?
    concentric/eccentric

Score: ___/9

MUSCLE STABILIZATIONS

Circle the letter of the best answer to the question.

1. Which of the following muscles can stabilize the wrist joint?
   a. Extensor digitorum
   b. Flexor digitorum profundus
   c. Abductor pollicis longus
   d. All of the above

2. Which of the following muscles can stabilize the saddle joint of the thumb?
   a. Abductor pollicis longus
   b. Extensor pollicis brevis
   c. Extensor pollicis longus
   d. All of the above

3. Which of the following muscles can stabilize the radioulnar joints?
   a. Extensor digitorum
   b. Supinator
   c. Extensor digiti minimi
   d. Flexor digitorum superficialis

4. Which of the following muscles can stabilize finger joints two through five?
   a. Extensor digitorum
   b. Brachioradialis
   c. Abductor pollicis longus
   d. Extensor carpi ulnaris

Score: ___/4

YOU'VE GOT NERVE!

Write in the name of the corresponding innervation from the list provided. Choices can be used more than once.

Median nerve

Ulnar nerve

Radial nerve

1. Extensor carpi radialis longus _____

2. Extensor carpi ulnaris _____

3. Extensor digitorum _____

4. Abductor pollicis longus _____

5. Abductor pollicis brevis _____

6. Extensor indicis _____

Score: ___/6

ARE YOU FEELING IT? – PALPATION

Fill in the blank with the best answer to the palpation question.

1. What muscle is palpated by pinching the radial group away from the forearm and then sinking down between the radial group and extensor digitorum? _____

2. What muscle is palpated immediately posterior to the shaft of the ulna?

111

3. What joint action should the client engage as you palpate the extensors carpi radialis longus and brevis? _____

_____

4. When adding resistance to the palpation protocol for the extensor carpi radialis muscles, where should you apply the resistance? _____

5. What muscle is palpated in the middle of the posterior forearm with the client extending the fingers at the metacarpophalangeal and interphalangeal joints?

_____

Score: ___/5

CLINICALLY SPEAKING

Fill in the blank with the best answer for the treatment consideration question.

1. Overuse of the wrist extensor group would likely cause what condition?

_____

2. What extensor muscle in the posterior forearm engages to stabilize the wrist joint from flexing when the fingers are flexed? _____

3. What nerve runs through the supinator and can become entrapped?

_____

4. The distal tendons of what two muscles are involved in de Quervain's disease?

_____

5. Flexor carpi ulnaris often blends with what other two muscles?

_____

Score: ___/5

MUSCLE MASH-UP

Fill in the blank with the best answer to the question.

1. What are the names of the three muscles of the wrist extensor group? _____

_____

2. Where does the common extensor tendon attach? _____

3. Where does the common flexor tendon attach? _____

4. How are the flexor carpi ulnaris and extensor carpi ulnaris synergistic to each other?

_____

5. How are the flexor carpi ulnaris and extensor carpi ulnaris antagonistic to each other?

_____

6. What are the names of the three thumb muscles of the deep distal four group?

_____

7. Excluding the thumb, which two fingers of the hand have two extensor muscles?

_____

8. What is the common name for lateral epicondylitis? _____

9. Name two muscles that attach to the lateral supracondylar ridge of the humerus.

_____

10. What bone is palpated in the anatomic snuffbox? _____

11. Friction against what bony landmark causes de Quervain's disease?

_____

12. What muscle's distal aponeurotic expansion is called the dorsal digital expansion?

_____

13. The distal tendons of what two deep distal four muscles are directly next to each other?

_____

14. The brachioradialis is superficial for its entire course except for the tendons of which two muscles that overlie it in the distal forearm?

_____

15. What muscle is deep in the proximal posterior forearm? _____

Score: ___/15

MINI CASE STUDIES

Fill in the blank with the best answer for the clinical case study questions.

1. A client has been referred to you for therapy of tennis elbow. Where on the client should you work?

_____

_____

2. What muscles are important to assess and possibly work in a client who has de Quervain's disease? _____

_____

3. What condition do you suspect if the client has pain with motion of the thumb and tenderness at the styloid process of the radius? _____

4. Which forearm extensor muscle would likely become tight from gripping the hand a lot?

_____

Score: ___/4

113

Use the clues to complete the crossword puzzle.

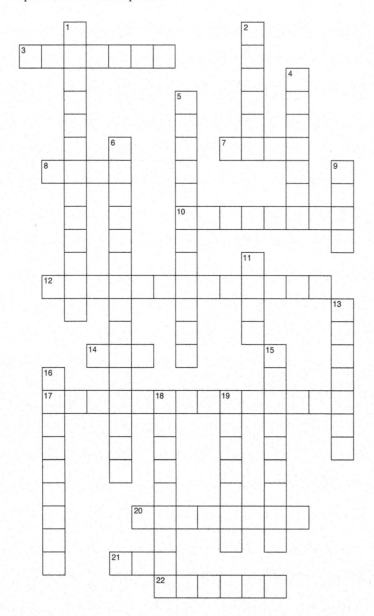

ACROSS

3 Bellies of extrinsic finger muscles are located here
7 The extensor carpi ulnaris also attaches to the _____
8 Number of distal tendons of the extensor digitorum
10 Lateral epicondylosis affects this common tendon
12 de Quervain's is this type of condition
14 Extensor muscle of little finger (acronym)
17 Engages the flexor carpi ulnaris (two words)
20 Thumb
21 This muscle is antagonistic to both actions of the extensor carpi radialis longus (acronym)
22 Location of common flexor tendon

DOWN

1 Antagonist to supinator (two words)
2 Nerve that innervates all posterior forearm muscles
4 Ulnar deviates
5 Digiti minimi (two words)
6 Attaches on humerus immediately proximal to the extensor carpi radialis longus
9 Extensor that contracts when fingers flex (acronym)
11 Number of muscles that attach into the common flexor tendon
13 The abductor pollicis longus abducts and _____
15 What are muscles that originate (attach proximally) outside of the hand and insert (attach distally) within the hand called?
16 Attaches to lateral epicondyle of humerus
18 The extensor digiti minimi often blends with this extensor muscle
19 Index finger

Score: ___/22

KNOW YOUR MUSCLES

Section 3 tests your knowledge of muscles covered in pages 222-236 of the *Know the Body* textbook.
Fill in the blank with the name of the muscles shown.

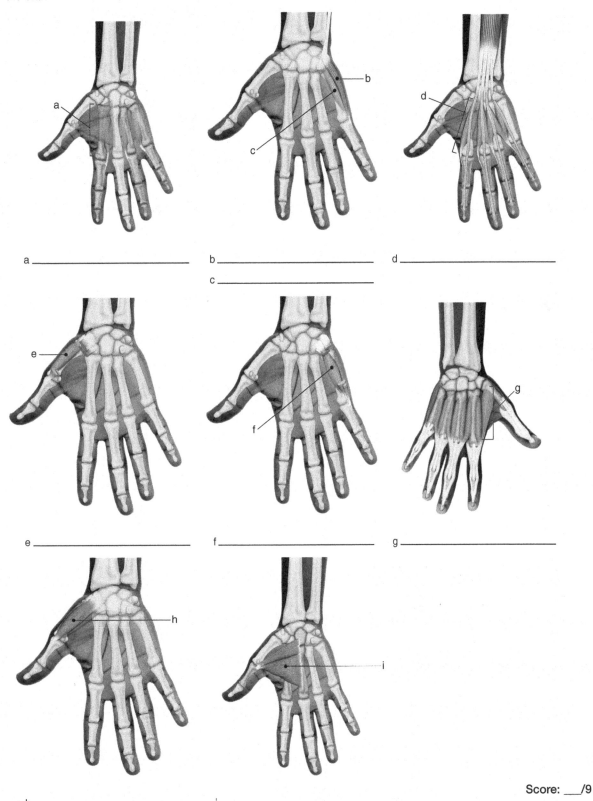

a _____

b _____

c _____

d _____

e _____

f _____

g _____

h _____

i _____

Score: ___/9

115

Match the muscle name from the right column to its meaning in the left column. Write your answer in the space provided. Each choice can be used only once.

Meaning

_____ 1. Opposes little finger

_____ 2. Shorter muscle that flexes the thumb

_____ 3. Flexes little finger

_____ 4. Between bones on palm side

_____ 5. Adducts thumb

_____ 6. Shorter muscle that attaches into the palm

_____ 7. Shorter muscle that abducts the thumb

_____ 8. Between bones on dorsal side of hand

_____ 9. Earthworm-shaped in the hand

_____ 10. Opposes the thumb

_____ 11. Abducts little finger

Muscle name

a. Flexor pollicis brevis

b. Flexor digiti minimi manus

c. Adductor pollicis

d. Dorsal interossei manus

e. Lumbricals manus

f. Palmar interossei

g. Opponens pollicis

h. Palmaris brevis

i. Abductor digiti minimi manus

j. Opponens digiti minimi

k. Abductor pollicis brevis

Score: ___/11

MATCHING ATTACHMENTS

Match each muscle from the word bank with its attachments. Write the answer in the column labeled *Muscle*. Each choice will be used only once.

Flexor pollicis brevis   Abductor digiti minimi manus

Lumbricals manus   Flexor digiti minimi manus

Adductor pollicis   Opponens pollicis

Opponens digiti minimi   Abductor pollicis brevis

Dorsal interossei manus   Palmaris brevis

Palmar interossei

Attachments	Muscle
1. The flexor retinaculum and the scaphoid and the trapezium *to the* Proximal phalanx of the thumb	
2. The flexor retinaculum and the trapezium *to the* Proximal phalanx of the thumb	
3. The flexor retinaculum and the trapezium *to the* First metacarpal (of the thumb)	
4. The pisiform *to the* Proximal phalanx of the little finger (finger 5)	
5. The flexor retinaculum and the hamate *to the* Proximal phalanx of the little finger (finger 5)	

116

6. The flexor retinaculum and the hamate *to the* Fifth metacarpal (of the little finger)	
7. The flexor retinaculum and the palmar aponeurosis *to the* Dermis of the ulnar (medial) border of the hand	
8. Third metacarpal and capitate *to the* Proximal phalanx of the thumb	
9. The distal tendons of the flexor digitorum profundus muscle *to the* Distal tendons of the extensor digitorum muscle (the dorsal digital expansion)	
10. The metacarpals of fingers 2, 4, and 5 *to the* Proximal phalanges of fingers 2, 4, and 5 on the "middle finger side"	
11. The metacarpals of fingers 1 through 5 *to the* Proximal phalanges of fingers 2, 3, and 4 on the side that faces away from the center of the middle finger	

Score: ___/11

THE BIG PICTURE – FUNCTIONAL GROUPS

Fill in the blanks with 1) the direction of movement, 2) the body part that is moving, and 3) the joint at which movement is occurring.

1. If a muscle crosses the metacarpophalangeal joints of fingers 2 through 5 anteriorly with a vertical direction to its fibers, what action can it perform?

   _____ of the _____ at the _____ joint(s).

2. If a muscle crosses the metacarpophalangeal joints of fingers 2 through 5 posteriorly with a vertical direction to its fibers, what action can it perform?

   _____ of the _____ at the _____ joint(s).

3. If a muscle attaches to the side of a finger that faces the middle finger, what action can it perform?

   _____ of the _____ at the _____ joint(s).

4. If a muscle attaches to the side of a finger that faces away from the middle finger, what action can it perform?

   _____ of the _____ at the _____ joint(s).

5. If a muscle crosses the carpometacarpal joint of the thumb on the anterior side, what action can it perform?

   _____ of the _____ at the _____ joint(s).

6. If a muscle crosses the carpometacarpal joint of the thumb on the posterior side, what action can it perform?

_____ of the _____ at the _____ joint(s).

7. If a muscle crosses the carpometacarpal joint of the thumb on the lateral side, what action can it perform?

_____ of the _____ at the _____ joint(s).

8. If a muscle crosses the carpometacarpal joint of the thumb on the medial side, what action can it perform?

_____ of the _____ at the _____ joint(s).

Score: ___/8

MATCHING ACTIONS

Place the corresponding joint action letter(s) in the blank(s) next to the muscle. The number of blanks next to each muscle name indicates the number of letters that should be placed next to that muscle.

Note: Fingers 2 through 5 move at the metacarpophalangeal, proximal interphalangeal, and distal interphalangeal joints; and the thumb at the saddle, metacarpophalangeal, and interphalangeal joints.

Joint Action

a. Flexes fingers 2 through 5

b. Flexes finger 5

c. Abducts fingers 2 through 4

d. Abducts finger 5

e. Abducts fingers 2, 4, and 5

f. Flexes the thumb

g. Abducts the thumb

h. Adducts the thumb

i. Opposes the thumb

j. Opposes finger 5

k. Wrinkles the skin of the palm

Muscle

1. Abductor pollicis brevis ____

2. Flexor pollicis brevis ____

3. Opponens pollicis ____

4. Abductor digiti minimi manus ____

5. Flexor digiti minimi manus ____

6. Opponens digiti minimi ____

7. Palmaris brevis ____

8. Adductor pollicis ____

9. Lumbricals manus ____

10. Palmar interossei ____

11. Dorsal interossei manus ____

Score: ___/11

THE LONG AND THE SHORT OF IT – EXERCISE 1

For each joint action given, indicate whether the muscle shortens or lengthens.

1. Abductor pollicis brevis: abduction of the thumb: _____

2. Flexor pollicis brevis: extension of the thumb: _____

3. Abductor digiti minimi manus: adduction of the little finger: _____

4. Adductor pollicis: adduction of the thumb: _____

5. Dorsal interossei manus: adduction of fingers 2 through 5: _____

118

Score: ___/5

THE LONG AND THE SHORT OF IT – EXERCISE 2

For each joint action given, fill in the blanks with a muscle that shortens and a muscle that lengthens. Please note that possible answers may be covered in another section or chapter.

1. Adduction of the thumb:

   Shortens: _____   Lengthens: _____

2. Abduction of the thumb:

   Shortens: _____   Lengthens: _____

3. Adduction of the index finger:

   Shortens: _____   Lengthens: _____

4. Abduction of the little finger:

   Shortens: _____   Lengthens: _____

5. Extension of the little finger:

   Shortens: _____   Lengthens: _____

Score: ___/10

MOVERS & ANTAGONISTS – EXERCISE 1

For each joint action stated, fill in the blank for a mover and antagonist of that joint action. Please choose your mover/antagonist pairs from the word bank below. Each pair can be used only once.

   Flexor pollicis brevis/Extensor pollicis longus

   Extensor digitorum/Flexor digitorum profundus

   Adductor pollicis/Abductor pollicis brevis

   Palmar interossei/Dorsal interossei manus

1. Adduction of fingers at the metacarpophalangeal joints:

   _____

2. Adduction of the thumb at the carpometacarpal joint:

   _____

3. Flexion of the thumb at the carpometacarpal joint:

   _____

4. Extension of fingers 2 through 5 at the metacarpophalangeal joints:

   _____

Score: ___/4

MUSCLE STABILIZATIONS

Circle the letter of the best answer to the question.

1. Which of the following muscles can stabilize the saddle joint of the thumb?
   a. Abductor pollicis brevis
   b. Flexor pollicis brevis
   c. Opponens pollicis
   d. All of the above

2. Which of the following muscles can stabilize the metacarpophalangeal joint of the little finger?
   a. Adductor pollicis
   b. Dorsal interossei manus
   c. Palmaris brevis
   d. Abductor digiti minimi manus

3. Which of the following muscles can stabilize the metacarpophalangeal joints of fingers 2 through 5?
   a. Flexor pollicis brevis
   b. Lumbricals manus
   c. Opponens digiti minimi
   d. All of the above

Score: ___/3

YOU'VE GOT NERVE!

Write in the name of the corresponding innervation(s) from the list provided. Choices will be used more than once.

Median nerve

Ulnar nerve

Radial nerve

1. Abductor pollicis brevis _____

2. Opponens pollicis _____ & _____

3. Flexor digiti minimi _____

4. Opponens digiti minimi _____

5. Adductor pollicis _____

6. Lumbricals manus _____ & _____

Score: ___/8

ARE YOU FEELING IT? – PALPATION

Fill in the blank with the best answer to the palpation question.

1. Where is the adductor pollicis palpated? _____

2. What intrinsic muscle of the hand is palpated by curling your finger pads around the metacarpal of the thumb?

   _____

3. What intrinsic muscle of the hand is palpated on the medial side of the thenar eminence? _____

   _____

4. What intrinsic muscle on the palmar side of the hand is palpated by placing a pen or highlighter between the fingers?

_____

5. What intrinsic muscle of the hand is palpated on the medial side of the hypothenar eminence?

_____

Score: ___/5

CLINICALLY SPEAKING

Fill in the blank with the best answer for the treatment consideration question.

1. The increased use of cell phones has led to this newly named condition.

_____

2. What name is given to osteoarthritis (degenerative joint disease) of the saddle joint of the thumb?

_____

3. Engagement of what intrinsic muscle of the hand can be used to engage and palpate the flexor carpi ulnaris?

_____

4. Which two intrinsic muscles of the hand usually have sesamoid bones located within their distal tendons?

_____

5. Which dorsal interosseus manus is the largest? _____

Score: ___/5

MUSCLE MASH-UP

Fill in the blank with the best answer to the question.

1. What are the names of the three muscles of the thenar group?

_____

2. What are the names of the three muscles of the hypothenar group?

_____

3. What are the four muscles/muscle groups of the central compartment group?

_____

4. Which muscle of the thenar eminence group is the most superficial?

_____

5. Why is the word "brevis" part of the muscle name "flexor pollicis brevis"?

_____

Chapter **7** **Muscles of the Forearm and Hand**

6. What is a common fascial attachment for all three muscles of the thenar eminence group?

_____

7. What is the only thenar eminence muscle that does not cross the metacarpophalangeal joint?

_____

8. Which muscle of the hypothenar eminence group is the deepest?

_____

9. Why is the word "manus" part of the muscle name "abductor digiti minimi manus"?

_____

10. What intrinsic hand muscle attaches to the pisiform?

_____

11. What thin fascial muscle overlies the hypothenar group?

_____

12. What intrinsic hand muscles are palpated on the dorsal side of the hand?

_____

13. Attaches from the tendons of one muscle to the tendons of another muscle.

_____

14. Other than the thumb, the palmar interossei do not attach to this finger.

_____

15. Other than the thumb, the dorsal interossei manus do not attach to this finger.

_____

Score: ___/15

CROSSWORD PUZZLE

Use the clues to complete the crossword puzzle.

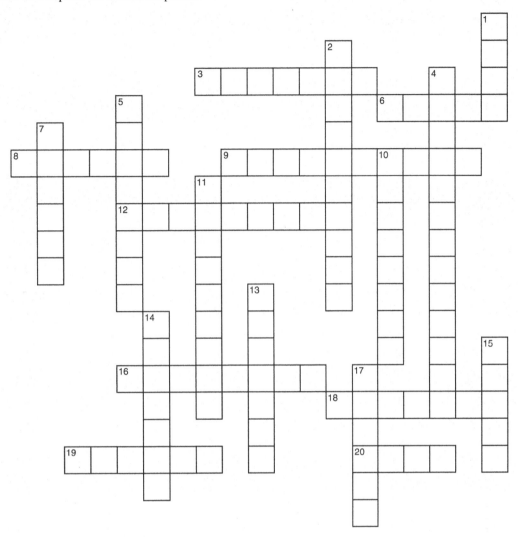

ACROSS

3 Adductor pollicis head
6 Innervation of hypothenar muscles
8 Reference line for abduction-adduction goes through this finger
9 Means "between bones"
12 Originates and inserts in the hand
16 Majority of the thumb web is composed of this "pollicis" muscle
18 Arthritis of saddle joint of thumb
19 Principal innervation of thenar muscles
20 Can also oppose their thumb

DOWN

1 Number of dorsal interossei manus
2 Intrinsic hand muscles palpated with the MCP joint flexed and IP joints extended
4 For lumbricals, palpate here on a metacarpal
5 Thumb
7 Third palmar interosseus is palpated between metacarpals of ring and what other finger?
10 Flexor pollicis brevis and adductor pollicis each have one
11 Carpal bone attachment for all thenar eminence muscles
13 Pathologic condition: _____ thumb
14 The first dorsal interosseus is also known as the abductor _____
15 Number of palmar interossei
17 Opponens digiti minimi attaches to this carpal

Score: ___/20

MINI CASE STUDIES

Fill in the blank with the best answer for the treatment consideration question.

1. A client comes to you because of pain in the thumb web. What muscles should you assess and likely work?

_____

2. You caution a client of yours who is constantly using her cell phone that she may develop this arthritic condition.

_____

3. A new client states that she uses her cell phone for emailing and texting a lot. What muscles are important to assess?

_____

_____

4. A fellow manual therapist comes to you with pain in and around the little finger. You decide to assess what muscle group. _____

Score: ___/4

MNEMONICS

Create your own mnemonic for the muscle group.

Wrist flexor group:

Flexor Carpi Radialis, Palmaris Longus, Flexor Carpi Ulnaris

Five Cats Ran Past Lucy's Favorite Crystal Unicorn

Now make one of your own:

F _____ C_____ R _____ P _____ L _____

F _____ C _____ U _____.

Wrist extensor group:

Extensor Carpi Radialis Longus, Extensor Carpi Radialis Brevis, Extensor Carpi Ulnaris

Every Child Respects Love, Every Child Respects Bravery, Every Child Understands

Now make one of your own:

E _____ C _____ R _____ L _____ E _____

C _____ R _____ B _____ E _____ C _____ U _____.

Radial Group:

Brachioradialis, Extensor Carpi Radialis Longus, Extensor Carpi Radialis Brevis

Because Every Child Receives Love, Every Child Relates Better.

Now make one of your own:

B _____ E _____ C _____ R _____ L _____

E _____ C _____ R _____ B _____ .

Thenar Group:

Abductor Pollicis Brevis, Flexor Pollicis Brevis, Opponens Pollicis

A Perfect Boy Friend Pleases By Offering Presents!

Now make one of your own:

A _____ P _____ B _____ F _____ P_____

B _____ O _____ P _____ .

Hypothenar Group:

Flexor Digiti Minimi Manus, ABductor Digiti Minimi Manus, Opponens Digiti Minimi

Find Da Money Mugsy, And Bring Da Money Mugsy, On Dis Monday! (said with a 1940s New York accent ☺)

Now make one of your own:

F _____ D _____ M _____ M _____

A _____ B _____ D _____ M _____ M _____

O _____ D _____ M _____ .

Central Compartment:

Adductor Pollicis, Lumbricals Manus, Palmar Interossei, Dorsal Interossei Manus

Algebra Pleases Lizzy's Math Professor, It Doesn't Interest Me!

Now make one of your own:

A_____P_____L_____M_____P_____I_____

D _____ I _____ M _____ .

Interossei Muscles' Actions:

Dorsal ABduct - Palmar ADduct

DAB - PAD

Now make one of your own:

D _____ AB _____ P _____ AD _____ .

Chapter **7 Muscles of the Forearm and Hand**

Muscles of the Spine and Rib Cage

COLORING & LABELING

Use crayons or felt-tipped markers to color the muscles. Use the word banks to fill in the numbers that correspond to the names of the muscles, bones, and bony landmarks in the blanks provided.

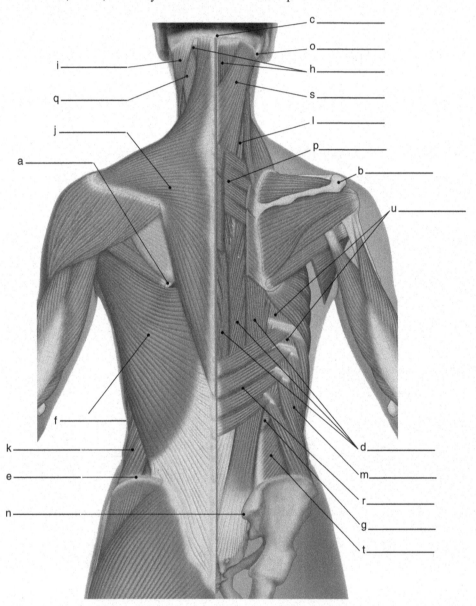

1. Acromion process of scapula
2. Erector spinae group
3. External abdominal oblique
4. External abdominal oblique
5. External intercostals

6. External occipital protuberance
7. Iliac crest
8. Inferior angle of scapula
9. Internal abdominal oblique
10. Latissimus dorsi

11. Mastoid process of temporal bone
12. Posterior superior iliac spine
13. Semispinalis capitis
14. Serratus posterior inferior
15. Serratus posterior superior

16. Splenius capitis
17. Splenius capitis
18. Splenius cervicis
19. Sternocleidomastoid
20. Transversus abdominis
21. Trapezius

Score: ___/21

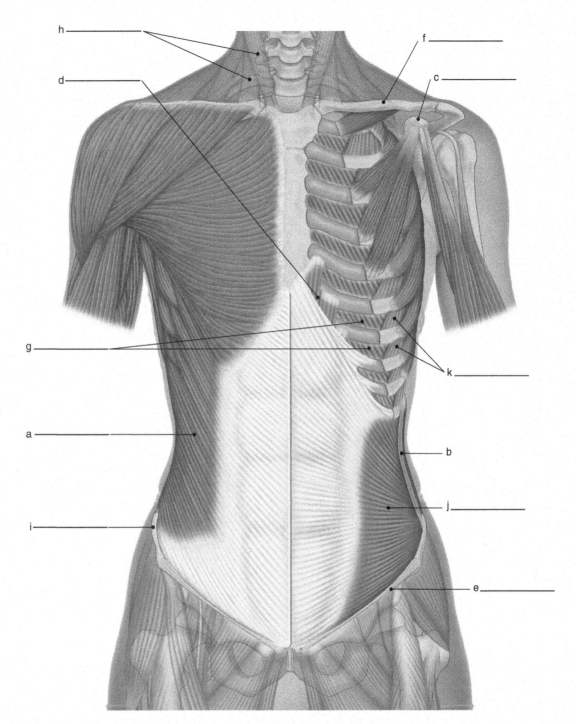

h _____

f _____

d _____

c _____

g _____

k _____

a _____

b _____

i _____

j _____

e _____

1. Clavicle
2. Coracoid process of scapula
3. External abdominal oblique

4. External abdominal oblique (cut)
5. External intercostals
6. Iliac crest

7. Inguinal ligament
8. Internal abdominal oblique
9. Internal intercostals

10. Rectus abdominis
11. Sternocleidomastoid

Score: ___/11

127

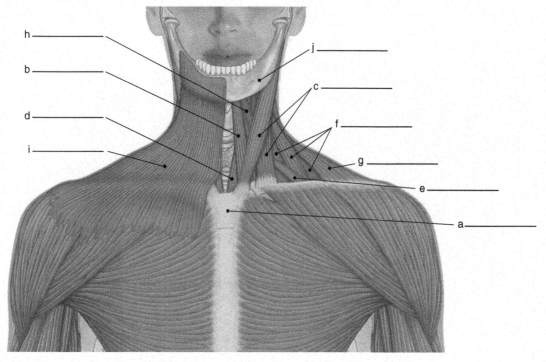

1. Mandible
2. Manubrium of sternum
3. Omohyoid
4. Omohyoid
5. Platysma
6. Scalenes
7. Sternocleidomastoid
8. Sternohyoid
9. Sternothyroid
10. Trapezius

Score: ___/10

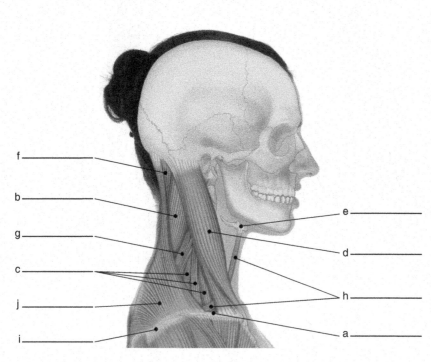

1. Acromion process of scapula
2. Clavicle
3. Hyoid bone
4. Levator scapulae
5. Omohyoid
6. Scalenes
7. Semispinalis capitis
8. Splenius capitis
9. Sternocleidomastoid
10. Trapezius

Score: ___/10

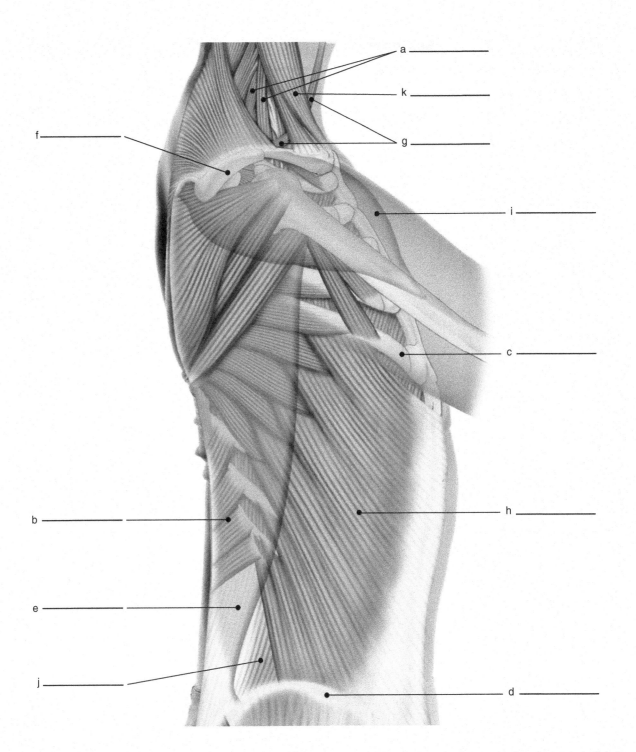

1. 5th rib
2. Acromion process of scapula
3. Deltoid
4. External abdominal oblique
5. Iliac crest
6. Internal abdominal oblique
7. Latissimus dorsi
8. Omohyoid
9. Scalenes
10. Serratus posterior inferior
11. Sternocleidomastoid

Score: ___/11

Section 1 tests your knowledge of muscles covered in pages 250–259 of the *Know the Body* textbook.

KNOW YOUR MUSCLES

Fill in the blank with the name of the muscles shown.

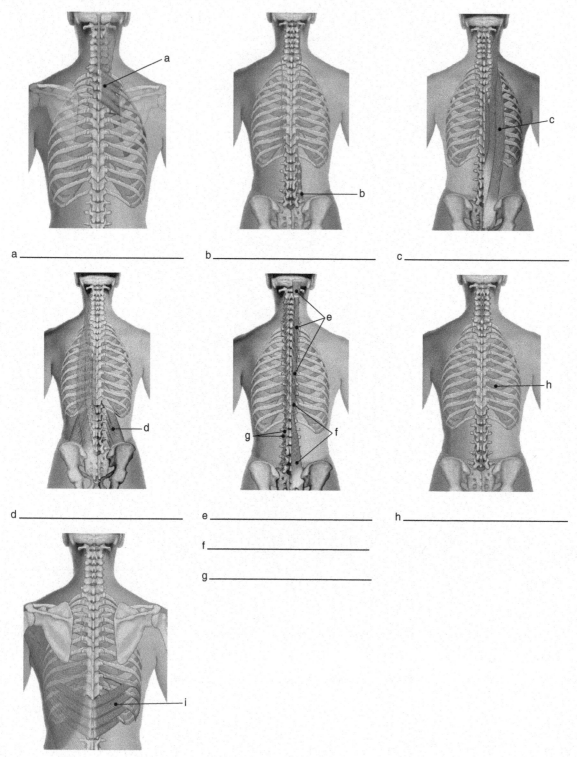

a _____

b _____

c _____

d _____

e _____

f _____

g _____

h _____

i _____

Score: ___/9

Chapter **8** **Muscles of the Spine and Rib Cage**

WHAT'S IN A NAME?

Match the muscle name from the right column to its meaning in the left column. Write your answer in the space provided. Each choice can be used only once.

Meaning

_____ 1. Squared muscle of the lumbar region

_____ 2. Notched muscle of the upper back

_____ 3. Between the transverse processes

_____ 4. Notched muscle of the lower back

_____ 5. To erect the spine

_____ 6. From transverse process to spinous process

_____ 7. Between the spinous processes

Muscle name

a. Transversospinalis

b. Serratus posterior superior

c. Serratus posterior inferior

d. Quadratus Lumborum

e. Interspinales

f. Intertransversarii

g. Erector spinae

Score: ___/7

MATCHING ATTACHMENTS

Match each muscle from the word bank with its attachments. Write the answer in the column labeled *Muscle*. Each choice will be used only once.

Quadratus lumborum   Interspinales

Erector Spinae   Intertransversarii

Serratus posterior superior   Serratus posterior inferior

Transversospinalis

Attachment	Muscle
1. Pelvis *to the* Spine, rib cage, and mastoid process of the temporal bone	
2. Pelvis and transverse processes of the spine *to the* Spinous processes of the spine, and the head	
3. Spinous process *to the* Spinous process directly superior	
4. Transverse process *to the* Transverse process directly superior	
5. Spinous processes of C7-T3 *to* Ribs 2 through 5	

6. Spinous processes of T11-L2
   to
   Ribs 9 through 12	

7. 12th rib and the transverse processes of L1-L4
   to the
   Posterior iliac crest	

Score: ___/7

THE BIG PICTURE – FUNCTIONAL GROUPS

Fill in the blanks with 1) the direction of movement, 2) the body part that is moving, and 3) the joint at which movement is occurring.

1. If a muscle crosses the spinal joints of the trunk posteriorly with a vertical direction to its fibers, what action can it perform?

   _____ of the _____ at the _____ joint(s).

2. If a muscle crosses the spinal joints of the trunk anteriorly with a vertical direction to its fibers, what action can it perform?

   _____ of the _____ at the _____ joint(s).

3. If a muscle crosses the spinal joints of the trunk laterally with a vertical direction to its fibers, what action can it perform?

   _____ of the _____ at the _____ joint(s).

4. If a muscle attaches to the pelvis and its other attachment is superior to the pelvic attachment, what action can it perform?

   _____ of the _____ at the _____ joint(s).

5. If a muscle attaches to the rib cage and its other attachment is superior to the rib cage attachment, what action can it perform?

   _____ of the _____ at the _____ joint(s).

6. If a muscle attaches to the rib cage and its other attachment is inferior to the rib cage attachment, what action can it perform?

   _____ of the _____ at the _____ joint(s).

7. What is the reverse action of extension of the upper spine relative to the lower spine?

   _____

Score: ___/7

MATCHING ACTIONS

Place the corresponding joint action letter(s) in the blank(s) next to the muscle. The number of blanks next to each muscle name indicates the number of letters that should be placed next to that muscle. Choices can be used more than once.

Joint Action

a. Extends the trunk

b. Extends the neck and trunk

c. Extends the trunk, neck, and head

d. Laterally flexes the trunk

e. Laterally flexes the neck and trunk

f. Laterally flexes the neck, trunk, and head

g. Contralaterally rotates the trunk and neck

h. Anteriorly tilts the pelvis

i. Elevates ribs 2 through 5

j. Depresses ribs 9 through 12

k. Depresses the 12th rib

l. Elevates the same-side pelvis

Muscle

1. Erector spinae ____ ____ ____

2. Transversospinalis ____ ____ ____ ____

3. Interspinales ____

4. Intertransversarii ____

5. Serratus posterior superior ____

6. Serratus posterior inferior ____

7. Quadratus lumborum ____ ____ ____ ____ ____

Score: ___/16

THE LONG AND THE SHORT OF IT – EXERCISE 1

For each joint action given, indicate whether the muscle shortens or lengthens.

1. Quadratus lumborum: elevation of the 12th rib: _____

2. Erector spinae: extension of the neck: _____

3. Interspinales: extension of the trunk: _____

4. Serratus posterior superior: depression of ribs 2 through 5:_____

5. Transversospinalis: ipsilateral rotation of the trunk: _____

Score: ___/5

THE LONG AND THE SHORT OF IT – EXERCISE 2

For each joint action given, fill in the blanks with a muscle that shortens and a muscle that lengthens. Please note that possible answers may be covered in another section.

1. Joint Action: extension of the trunk

    Shortens: _____   Lengthens: _____

2. Joint Action: anterior tilt of the pelvis

    Shortens: _____   Lengthens: _____

3. Joint Action: posterior tilt of the pelvis

    Shortens: _____   Lengthens: _____

4. Joint Action: depression of the ribs

    Shortens: _____   Lengthens: _____

5. Joint Action: flexion of the neck

    Shortens: _____   Lengthens: _____

Score: ___/10

MOVERS & ANTAGONISTS – EXERCISE 1

For each joint action stated, fill in the blank for a mover and antagonist of that joint action. Please choose your mover/antagonist pairs from the word bank below. Each pair can be used only once.

Serratus posterior superior/Serratus posterior inferior

Right iliocostalis/Left longissimus

Left rotatores/Right rotatores

1. Elevates the ribs at sternocostal and costospinal joints:

    _____

2. Right rotation of the trunk at the spinal joints:

    _____

3. Right lateral flexion of the trunk at the spinal joints:

    _____

Score: ___/3

For each joint action illustrated, the body part is being *slowly* moved in the direction indicated by the arrow. Circle whether the functional muscle group of the pair provided is contracting or relaxed. Then circle *how* the muscle group that is working is contracting (concentrically or eccentrically).

1.

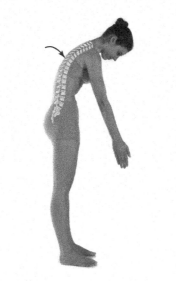

Movement:

Flexion of the trunk at the spinal joints

Flexors: contracting/relaxed

Extensors: contracting/relaxed

What type of contraction is occurring?
concentric/eccentric

2.

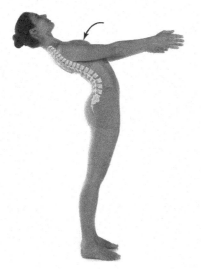

Movement:

Extension of the trunk at the spinal joints

Extensors: contracting/relaxed

Flexors: contracting/relaxed

What type of contraction is occurring?
concentric/eccentric

3.

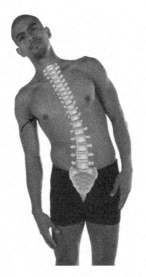

Movement:

Right lateral flexion of the trunk at the spinal joints

Right lateral flexors: contracting/relaxed

Left lateral flexors: contracting/relaxed

What type of contraction is occurring?
concentric/eccentric

Score: ___/9

Chapter **8** **Muscles of the Spine and Rib Cage**

MUSCLE STABILIZATIONS

Circle the letter of the best answer to the question.

1. Which of the following muscles can stabilize the 12th rib?
   a. Serratus posterior superior
   b. Interspinales
   c. Intertransversarii
   d. Quadratus lumborum

2. Which of the following muscles stabilizes the ribs at the sternocostal joints?
   a. Spinalis
   b. Transversospinalis
   c. Serratus posterior superior
   d. Quadratus lumborum

3. Which of the following muscle pairs stabilizes the sacroiliac joints?
   a. Serratus posterior inferior/Erector spinae
   b. Serratus posterior inferior/Interspinales
   c. Erector spinae/Transversospinalis
   d. Intertransversarii/Transversospinalis

4. Which of the following muscles does NOT stabilize lumbar spinal joints?
   a. Erector spinae
   b. Serratus posterior superior
   c. Transversospinalis
   d. Interspinales

Score: ___/4

YOU'VE GOT NERVE!

Write the name of the corresponding innervation(s) from the list provided. Choices can be used more than once.

Spinal nerves

Intercostal nerves

Subcostal nerve

Lumbar plexus

1. Erector spinae _____

2. Transversospinales _____

3. Interspinales _____

4. Intertransversarii _____

5. Serratus posterior superior _____

6. Serratus posterior inferior _____ & _____

7. Quadratus lumborum _____

Score: ___/7

ARE YOU FEELING IT? – PALPATION

Fill in the blank with the best answer to the palpation question.

1. What muscle is accessed when palpating deep and medial to the lateral border of the erector spinae in the lumbar region? _____

2. What actions should you ask the client to perform in order to palpate the transversospinalis musculature?

   _____

3. What muscle group is best engaged and palpated with extension of the trunk? _____

4. Where should you place your fingers to palpate the interspinales? _____

Score: ___/4

CLINICALLY SPEAKING

Fill in the blank with the best answer for the treatment consideration question.

1. What effect does tight erector spinae musculature have upon the lumbar spinal curve?

   _____

2. Name a muscle that is important for core stabilization of the spine.

   _____

3. What can happen to the posture of the pelvis if the quadratus lumborum is tight on one side?

   _____

4. This muscle group is important for guiding our descent as we bend forward.

   _____

Score: ___/4

MUSCLE MASH-UP

Fill in the blank with the best answer to the question.

1. Name the three subgroups of the erector spinae group. _____

2. Name the three subgroups of the transversospinalis group. _____

3. The _____ muscle attaches to the spine and depresses ribs 9 through 12.

4. The serratus posterior inferior is deep the _____ muscle.

5. In which two regions of the spine are the interspinales and intertransversarii located? _____

6. What is the most superior attachment of the erector spinae group? _____

Chapter **8 Muscles of the Spine and Rib Cage**

7. What muscle of the rib cage is deep to the trapezius and rhomboids? _____

8. What square-shaped muscle is deep to the erector spinae? _____

9. What is the deepest subgroup of the transversospinalis group? _____

10. What is the most lateral subgroup of the erector spinae group? _____

Score: ___/10

MINI CASE STUDIES

Fill in the blank with the best answer for the clinical case study questions.

1. A client presents with low back pain, a result of excessive bending of the trunk during their daily routine at work. What musculature do you assess first? _____

2. A person has a high iliac crest with a compensatory scoliosis. What muscle do you assess first?

_____

3. If a client presents with an excessive anteriorly tilted pelvis, what low back musculature do you look to assess first?

_____

Score: ___/3

CROSSWORD PUZZLE

Use the clues to complete the crossword puzzle.

ACROSS

5 Largest muscle in the neck
11 Between transverse processes
12 Like a knife

DOWN

1 Erector spinae and transversospinalis together
2 Important muscle for core stabilization
3 The erector spinae attaches inferiorly to this fascia
4 Transversospinalis: TP to _____
6 The transversospinalis can stabilize this joint
7 Square-shaped
8 Deep in the laminar groove
9 This posterior serratus muscle stabilizes the rib cage against the pull of the diaphragm
10 Serratus posterior inferior attaches to ribs nine through _____

Score: ___/12

Chapter **8 Muscles of the Spine and Rib Cage**

Section 2 tests your knowledge of muscles covered in pages 260–272 of the *Know the Body* textbook.

KNOW YOUR MUSCLES

Fill in the blank with the name of the muscles shown.

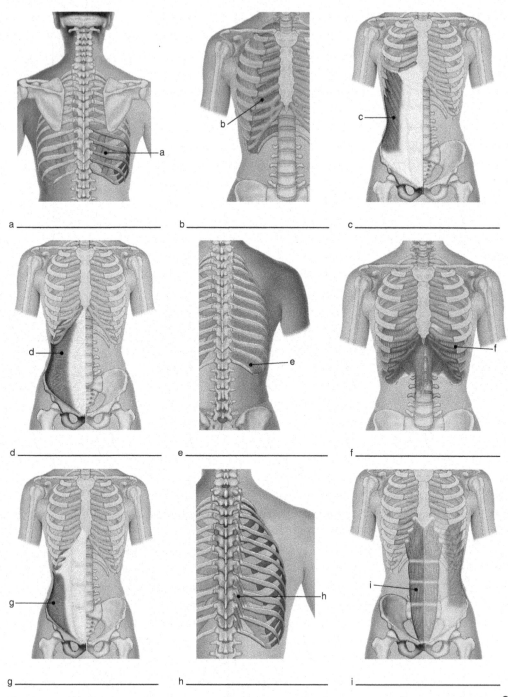

a _____

b _____

c _____

d _____

e _____

f _____

g _____

h _____

i _____

Score: ___/9

WHAT'S IN A NAME?

Match the muscle name from the right column to its meaning in the left column. Write your answer in the space provided. Each choice can be used only once.

Meaning

_____ 1. Superficial, abdomen, oblique angle

_____ 2. Superficial between the ribs

_____ 3. A partition

_____ 4. Under (or deep to) the ribs

_____ 5. Deeper between the ribs

_____ 6. Deep, abdomen, oblique angle

_____ 7. Elevator of the ribs

_____ 8. Transverse across the abdomen

_____ 9. Transverse across the thoracic region

_____ 10. Straight up the abdomen

Muscle name/term

a. Rectus abdominis

b. Transversus abdominis

c. Transversus thoracis

d. Internal abdominal oblique

e. Levatores costarum

f. External abdominal oblique

g. External intercostals

h. Diaphragm

i. Subcostales

j. Internal intercostals

Score: ___/10

MATCHING ATTACHMENTS

Match each muscle from the word bank with its attachments. Write the answer in the column labeled *Muscle*. Each choice can be used only once.

Subcostales   Transversus thoracis   Diaphragm

Levatores costarum   External intercostals   Rectus abdominis

Transversus abdominis   Internal abdominal obliques   Internal intercostals

External abdominal obliques

Attachments	Muscle name
1. In the intercostal spaces of ribs 1 through 12	
2. In the intercostal spaces of ribs 1 through 12	
3. Transverse processes of C7-T11 *to* Ribs 1 through 12	
4. Ribs 10 through 12 *to* Ribs 8 through 10	
5. Internal surfaces of the sternum, the xiphoid process, and the adjacent costal cartilages *to the* Internal surface of costal cartilages 2 through 6	

6. Inferior surfaces of the rib cage, sternum, and the spine
    to the
    Central tendon (dome) of the diaphragm	

7. Pubis
    to the
    Xiphoid process and the cartilage of ribs 5 through 7	

8. Anterior iliac crest, pubic bone, and the abdominal
    aponeurosis
    to the
    Lower eight ribs (ribs 5 through 12)	

9. Inguinal ligament, iliac crest, and the thoracolumbar
    fascia
    to the
    Lower three ribs (ribs 10 through 12) and the
    abdominal aponeurosis	

10. Inguinal ligament, iliac crest, thoracolumbar fascia,
    and the lower costal cartilages
    to the
    Abdominal aponeurosis	

Score: ___/10

THE BIG PICTURE – FUNCTIONAL GROUPS

Fill in the blanks with 1) the direction of movement, 2) the body part that is moving, and 3) the joint at which movement is occurring.

1. If a muscle crosses the spinal joints of the trunk anteriorly with a vertical direction to its fibers, what action can it perform?

   _____ of the _____ at the _____ joint(s).

2. If a muscle crosses the spinal joints of the trunk posteriorly with a vertical direction to its fibers, what action can it perform?

   _____ of the _____ at the _____ joint(s).

3. If a muscle crosses the spinal joints of the trunk laterally with a vertical direction to its fibers, what action can it perform?

   _____ of the _____ at the _____ joint(s).

4. If a muscle attaches to the pelvis anteriorly and its other attachment is superior to the pelvic attachment, what action can it perform?

   _____ of the _____ at the _____ joint(s).

5. If a muscle attaches to the rib cage and its other attachment is superior to the rib cage attachment, what action can it perform?

   _____ of the _____ at the _____ joint(s).

6. If a muscle attaches to the rib cage and its other attachment is inferior to the rib cage attachment, what action can it perform?

_____ of the _____ at the _____ joint(s).

7. What is the reverse action of flexion of the spine relative to the pelvis?

_____.

Score: ___/7

MATCHING ACTIONS

Place the corresponding joint action letter(s) in the blank(s) next to the muscle. The number of blanks next to each muscle name indicates the number of letters that should be placed next to that muscle.

Joint Action

a. Elevates the ribs

b. Depresses the ribs

c. Increases volume of the thoracic cavity

d. Compresses the abdominopelvic cavity

e. Flexes the trunk

f. Laterally flexes the trunk

g. Ipsilaterally rotates the trunk

h. Contralaterally rotates the trunk

i. Posteriorly tilts the pelvis

Muscle

1. External intercostals ___ ___

2. Internal intercostals ___ ___

3. Levatores costarum ___

4. Subcostales ___

5. Transversus thoracis ___

6. Diaphragm ___

7. Rectus abdominis ___ ___ ___

8. External abdominal obliques ___ ___ ___ ___

9. Internal abdominal obliques ___ ___ ___ ___

10. Transversus abdominis ___

Score: ___/20

THE LONG AND THE SHORT OF IT – EXERCISE 1

For each joint action given, indicate whether the muscle shortens or lengthens.

1. External intercostals: elevation of the ribs: _____

2. Rectus abdominis: flexion of the trunk: _____

3. Transversus abdominis: expansion of the abdominopelvic cavity: _____

4. Internal intercostals: contralateral rotation of the trunk: _____

5. Diaphragm: increasing the volume of the thoracic cavity: _____

Score: ___/5

143

THE LONG AND THE SHORT OF IT – EXERCISE 2

For each joint action given, fill in the blanks with a muscle that shortens and a muscle that lengthens. Please note that possible answers may be covered in another section.

1. Elevation of the ribs:

   Shortens: _____   Lengthens: _____

2. Depression of the ribs:

   Shortens: _____   Lengthens: _____

3. Contralateral rotation of the trunk:

   Shortens: _____   Lengthens: _____

4. Ipsilateral rotation of the trunk:

   Shortens: _____   Lengthens: _____

5. Flexion of the trunk:

   Shortens: _____   Lengthens: _____

Score: ___/10

MOVERS & ANTAGONISTS – EXERCISE 1

For each joint action stated, fill in the blank for a mover and antagonist of that joint action. Please choose your mover/antagonist pairs from the word bank below. Each pair can be used only once.

   Levatores costarum/Subcostales

   Rectus abdominis/Erector spinae group

   Left external abdominal oblique/Right internal abdominal oblique

   Left internal intercostals/Right internal intercostals

1. Flexes the trunk at the spinal joints:

   _____

2. Left rotation of the trunk at the spinal joints:

   _____

3. Elevates ribs at sternocostal and costospinal joints:

   _____

4. Left lateral flexion of the trunk at the spinal joints:

   _____

Score: ___/4

144

For each joint action illustrated, the body part is being *slowly* moved in the direction indicated by the arrow. Circle whether the functional muscle group of the pair provided is contracting or relaxed. Then circle *how* the muscle group that is working is contracting (concentrically or eccentrically).

1.

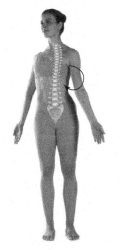

Movement:

Right lateral flexion of the trunk at the spinal joints

    Right lateral flexors: contracting/relaxed

    Left lateral flexors: contracting/relaxed

    What type of contraction is occurring?
    concentric/eccentric

2.

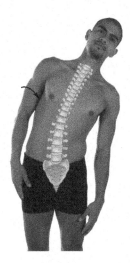

Movement:

Right rotation of the trunk at the spinal joints

    Right rotators: contracting/relaxed

    Left rotators: contracting/relaxed

    What type of contraction is occurring?
    concentric/eccentric

3.

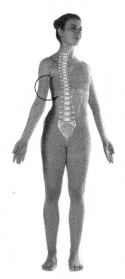

Movement:

Left rotation of the trunk at the spinal joints

    Left rotators: contracting/relaxed

    Right rotators: contracting/relaxed

    What type of contraction is occurring?
    concentric/eccentric

Score: ___/9

145

MUSCLE STABILIZATIONS

Circle the letter of the best answer to the question.

1. Which of the following muscles can stabilize the lumbar spinal joints, pelvis, and rib cage?
   a. Intercostales
   b. Transversus abdominis
   c. Diaphragm
   d. External intercostals

2. Which of the following muscles can stabilize the costospinal joints?
   a. Levatores costarum
   b. Transversus abdominis
   c. Subcostales
   d. All of the above

3. Which of the following muscles can stabilize the trunk, including the joints of the lower rib cage and the thoracic and lumbar spinal joints?
   a. External intercostals
   b. Transversus thoracis
   c. Diaphragm
   d. External abdominal oblique

4. Which of the following muscles best stabilizes the sternum?
   a. Diaphragm
   b. Intercostales
   c. Transversus abdominis
   d. Transversus thoracis

Score: ___/4

YOU'VE GOT NERVE!

Write the name of the corresponding innervation from the list provided. Choices can be used more than once.

Intercostal nerves

Spinal nerves

Phrenic nerve

1. External intercostals _____

2. Internal intercostals _____

3. Levatores costarum _____

4. Subcostales _____

5. Transversus thoracis _____

6. Diaphragm _____

7. Rectus abdominis _____

8. External abdominal oblique _____

9. Internal abdominal oblique _____

10. Transversus abdominis _____

Score: ___/10

ARE YOU FEELING IT? – PALPATION

Fill in the blank with the best answer to the palpation question.

1. What muscle of the anterior abdominal wall is palpated by asking the client to flex and contralaterally rotate the trunk?

   _____

2. What muscle is palpated on the internal surface of the rib cage as the client exhales?

   _____

3. In what region of the trunk can the intercostals be most easily accessed for palpation?

   _____

4. What muscle is palpated anteromedially in the trunk? _____

Score: ___/4

CLINICALLY SPEAKING

Fill in the blank with the best answer for the treatment consideration question.

1. What name is given to the fibrous bands that transect the rectus abdominis?

   _____

2. Although they're not the first muscle group we think of to help athletic function, working this muscle group to increase the body's oxygen intake is recommended with athletes. _____

3. What respiratory muscle is often held in isometric contraction when performing an activity that requires a great deal of strength? _____

4. Which attachment of the diaphragm moves during belly breathing?

   _____

Score: ___/4

MUSCLE MASH-UP

Fill in the blank with the best answer to the question.

1. What muscle is directly deep to the internal abdominal oblique?

   _____

2. What is considered to be the insertion (superior attachment) of the diaphragm?

   _____

3. What are the names of the abdominal oblique muscles?

   _____

147

4. What attaches from the transverse processes to ribs?

_____

5. What muscle group has the same fiber direction as the external abdominal oblique?

_____

6. Which are the four muscles of the anterior abdominal wall?

_____

7. This muscle attaches to the xiphoid process. _____

8. What is the sagittal plane action upon the pelvis of the rectus abdominis?

_____

9. To feel for the contraction of the transversus abdominis, ask the client to breathe _____.

10. To strum the rectus abdominis perpendicularly, in what direction do we strum?

_____

Score: ___/10

MINI CASE STUDIES

Fill in the blank with the best answer for the clinical case study questions.

1. If a client has poor core strength, which abdominal wall muscle(s) should they primarily strengthen?

_____

2. Strengthening what muscle group would help a client have a flat belly?

_____

3. What muscle group do you immediately assess for a client who presents with a chronic cough?

_____

4. Strengthening what muscle might help a client with a hiatal hernia?

_____

Score: ___/4

Use the clues to complete the crossword puzzle.

ACROSS

1 Pierces the diaphragm
5 Levator
6 Intercostals are involved with
   _____
9 Refers to ribs
10 Principal muscle of inspiration
11 The transversus abdominis
   acts like a _____

DOWN

2 Oriented diagonally
3 Deep to rib cage
4 Neck musculature that extends and
   ipsilaterally rotates
6 Straight
7 The three anterolateral abdominal wall
   muscles form the rectus _____
8 Spare rib meat

Score: ___/12

Section 3 tests your knowledge of muscles covered in pages 274–281 of the *Know the Body* textbook.

KNOW YOUR MUSCLES

Fill in the blank with the name of the muscles shown.

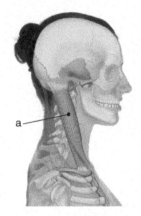

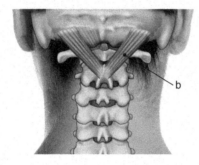

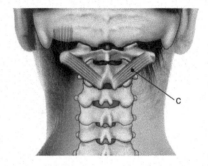

a _____

b _____

c _____

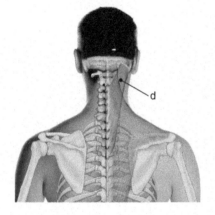

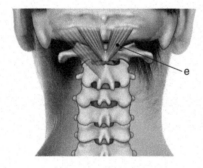

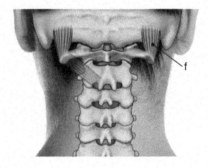

d _____

e _____

f _____

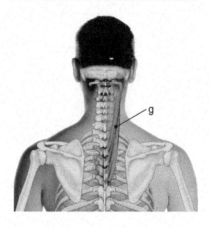

g _____

Score: ___/7

WHAT'S IN A NAME?

Match the muscle name from the right column to its meaning in the left column. Write your answer in the space provided. Each choice can be used only once.

Meaning

_____ 1. Muscle attaching to the sternum, clavicle, and the mastoid process

_____ 2. Larger, straighter muscle attached to the head

_____ 3. Smaller, straighter muscle attached to the head

_____ 4. Bandage-shaped muscle attached to the head

_____ 5. More inferiorly placed obliquely oriented muscle attaching on (or near) the head

_____ 6. Bandage-shaped muscle attached to the neck

_____ 7. More superiorly placed obliquely oriented muscle attaching on the head

Muscle name

a. Rectus capitis posterior major

b. Obliquus capitis superior

c. Splenius cervicis

d. Sternocleidomastoid

e. Rectus capitis posterior minor

f. Splenius capitis

g. Obliquus capitis inferior

Score: ___/7

MATCHING ATTACHMENTS

Match each muscle from the word bank with its attachments. Write the answer in the column labeled *Muscle*. Each choice can be used only once.

Splenius capitis   Rectus capitis posterior major   Obliquus capitis inferior

Splenius cervicis   Rectus capitis posterior minor   Obliquus capitis superior

Sternocleidomastoid

Attachments	Muscle
1. Nuchal ligament from C3-C6 and the spinous processes of C7-T4 *to the* Mastoid process of the temporal bone and the occipital bone	
2. Spinous processes of T3-T6 *to the* Transverse processes of C1-C3	
3. Spinous process of the Axis (C2) *to the* Occiput	
4. Posterior tubercle of the Atlas (C1) *to the* Occiput	

5. Spinous process of the Axis (C2) *to the* Transverse process of the Atlas (C1)	
6. Transverse process of the Atlas (C1) *to the* Occiput	
7. Sternal Head: Manubrium of the sternum Clavicular Head: Medial clavicle *to the* Mastoid process of the temporal bone	

Score: ___/7

THE BIG PICTURE – FUNCTIONAL GROUPS

Fill in the blanks with 1) the direction of movement, 2) the body part that is moving, and 3) the joint at which movement is occurring.

1. If a muscle crosses the spinal joints of the neck anteriorly with a vertical direction to its fibers, what action can it perform?

   _____ of the _____ at the _____ joint(s).

2. If a muscle crosses the spinal joints of the neck posteriorly with a vertical direction to its fibers, what action can it perform?

   _____ of the _____ at the _____ joint(s).

3. If a muscle crosses the spinal joints of the neck laterally on the right side with a vertical direction to its fibers, what action can it perform?

   _____ of the _____ at the _____ joint(s).

4. What is the reverse action of flexion of the upper spine relative to the lower spine?

   _____.

5. What is the reverse action of extension of the upper spine relative to the lower spine?

   _____.

Score: ___/5

MATCHING ACTIONS

Place the corresponding joint action letter(s) in the blank(s) next to the muscle. The number of blanks next to each muscle name indicates the number of letters that should be placed next to that muscle.

Joint Action

a. Extends the head at the atlanto-occipital joint

b. Protracts the head at the atlanto-occipital joint

c. Ipsilaterally rotates the atlas at the atlantoaxial joint

d. Extends the neck

Muscle

1. Splenius capitis ___ ___ ___

2. Splenius cervicis ___ ___ ___

e. Extends the head and neck

f. Extends the upper neck and head

g. Flexes the lower neck

h. Laterally flexes the neck

i. Laterally flexes the head and neck

j. Ipsilaterally rotates the neck

k. Ipsilaterally rotates the head and neck

l. Contralaterally rotates the head and neck

3. Rectus capitis posterior major ____

4. Rectus capitis posterior minor ____

5. Obliquus capitis inferior ____

6. Obliquus capitis superior ____

7. Sternocleidomastoid ____ ____ ____ ____

Score: ___/14

THE LONG AND THE SHORT OF IT – EXERCISE 1

For each joint action given, indicate whether the muscle shortens or lengthens.

1. Sternocleidomastoid: extension of the lower neck: _____

2. Splenius cervicis: ipsilateral rotation of the neck: _____

3. Splenius capitis: contralateral rotation of the head and neck:_____

4. Obliquus capitis superior: protraction of the head at the atlanto-occipital joint: _____

5. Rectus capitis posterior major: flexion of the head at the atlanto-occipital joint: _____

Score: ___/5

THE LONG AND THE SHORT OF IT – EXERCISE 2

For each joint action given, fill in the blanks with a muscle that shortens and a muscle that lengthens. Please note that possible answers may be covered in another section.

1. Extension of the neck:

   Shortens: _____   Lengthens: _____

2. Ipsilateral rotation the neck:

   Shortens: _____   Lengthens: _____

Chapter **8** **Muscles of the Spine and Rib Cage**

3. Contralateral rotation of the neck:

Shortens: _____   Lengthens: _____

4. Protraction of the head at the atlanto-occipital joint:

Shortens: _____

5. Flexion of the neck:

Shortens: _____   Lengthens: _____

Score: ___/10

MOVERS & ANTAGONISTS – EXERCISE 1

For each joint action stated, fill in the blank for a mover and antagonist of that joint action. Please choose your mover/antagonist pairs from the word bank below. Each pair can be used only once.

Right semispinalis capitis/Left upper trapezius

Right sternocleidomastoid/Right splenius capitis

Left sternocleidomastoid/Left splenius cervicis

1. Right rotation of the neck at the spinal joints:

_____

2. Flexes the neck at the spinal joints:

_____

3. Right lateral flexion of the neck at the spinal joints:

_____

Score: ___/3

For each joint action illustrated, the body part is being *slowly* moved in the direction indicated by the arrow. Circle whether the functional muscle group of the pair provided is contracting or relaxed. Then circle *how* the muscle group that is working is contracting (concentrically or eccentrically).

1.

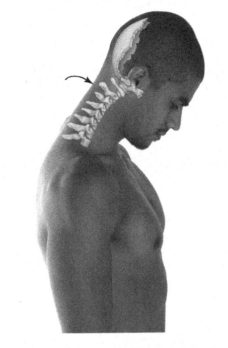

Movement:

Flexion of the neck at the spinal joints

   Flexors: contracting/relaxed

   Extensors: contracting/relaxed

   What type of contraction is occurring?
   concentric/eccentric

2.

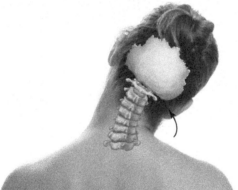

Movement:

Left lateral flexion of the neck at the spinal joints

   Left lateral flexors: contracting/relaxed

   Right lateral flexors: contracting/relaxed

   What type of contraction is occurring?
   concentric/eccentric

3.

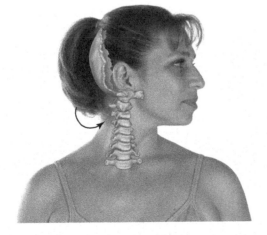

Movement:

Left rotation of the neck at the spinal joints

   Left rotators: contracting/relaxed

   Right rotators: contracting/relaxed

   What type of contraction is occurring?
   concentric/eccentric

Score: ___/9

155

MUSCLE STABILIZATIONS

Circle the letter of the best answer to the question.

1. Which of the following muscles can stabilize the cervical and upper thoracic vertebrae and the head?
   a. Splenius cervicis
   b. Splenius capitis
   c. Rectus capitis posterior minor
   d. Obliquus capitis superior

2. Which of the following muscles can stabilize the cervical and upper thoracic vertebrae?
   a. Rectus capitis posterior major
   b. Sternocleidomastoid
   c. Splenius cervicis
   d. Obliquus capitis inferior

3. Which of the following muscles stabilizes the head and atlas at the atlanto-occipital joint?
   a. Rectus capitis posterior major
   b. Obliquus capitis inferior
   c. Splenius cervicis
   d. Levator scapulae

4. Which of the following muscles can stabilize the atlantoaxial joint?
   a. Rectus capitis posterior minor
   b. Posterior scalene
   c. Obliquus capitis inferior
   d. Stylohyoid

Score: ___/4

YOU'VE GOT NERVE!

Write the name of the corresponding innervation from the list provided. Choices can be used more than once.

Cervical spinal nerves

Suboccipital nerve

Spinal accessory nerve (CN XI)

1. Splenius capitis _____

2. Splenius cervicis _____

3. Rectus capitis posterior major _____

4. Rectus capitis posterior minor _____

5. Obliquus capitis inferior _____

6. Obliquus capitis superior _____

7. Sternocleidomastoid _____

Score: ___/7

Fill in the blank with the best answer to the palpation question.

1. What muscle is palpated with the client supine and the neck rotated to the opposite side, and then the client lifts the head and neck toward the ceiling?

   _____

2. Where can the splenius capitis be found superficially?

   _____

3. What head of the sternocleidomastoid is usually more visible and palpable?

   _____

4. This muscle is used as a landmark to palpate the scalenes and longus muscles.

   _____

Score: ___/4

CLINICALLY SPEAKING

Fill in the blank with the best answer for the treatment consideration question.

1. These muscles function primarily as postural stabilizers of the head. _____

2. Working the sternocleidomastoid can affect blood pressure and requires caution due to the presence of what structure?

   _____

3. This muscle has a fascial connection to the dura mater. _____

4. What muscle forms the anterior border of the posterior triangle of the neck?

   _____

Score: ___/4

MUSCLE MASH-UP

Fill in the blank with the best answer to the question.

1. What are the names of the four suboccipital muscles?

   _____

2. What are the two splenius muscles?

   _____

3. Which splenius muscle is positioned deep?

   _____

4. Flexes the lower neck but extends the upper neck. _____

5. Suboccipital muscle whose primary action is ipsilateral rotation. _____

6. What are the two heads of the sternocleidomastoid?

_____

7. This muscle is located between the spinous process of C2 and the occiput. _____

8. What does capitis mean?

_____

9. What is the innervation of the sternocleidomastoid?

_____

10. Extends and ipsilaterally rotates the head. _____

Score: ___/10

MINI CASE STUDIES

Fill in the blank with the best answer for the clinical case study questions.

1. What condition might a client be experiencing if he has a tight rectus capitis posterior minor?

_____

2. A new client presents with an anteriorly held posture of the head. What muscles should be assessed?

_____

3. A client experienced a whiplash accident where his head was forcefully thrown back into extension. Which functional group of muscles were most likely injured?

_____

4. When you are working on a client's sternocleidomastoid and the client suddenly feels lightheaded and weak, what may have happened?

_____

Score: ___/4

CROSSWORD PUZZLE

Use the clues to complete the crossword puzzle.

ACROSS

3 Carotid _____
4 Smaller
5 Common car accident injury
7 Superficial muscle of neck
9 Both obliquus capitis muscles
   attach to this process of C1
11 Splenius capitis muscles known
   as (2 words)

DOWN

1 Abbreviation for sternocleidomastoid (acronym)
2 Carotid sinus reflex affects (2 words)
3 Bandage
6 Posterior _____
8 Larger
10 Obliquus capitis inferior crosses this joint (acronym)

Score: ___/12

Chapter **8   Muscles of the Spine and Rib Cage**

Section 4 tests your knowledge of muscles covered in pages 282–295 of the *Know the Body* textbook.

KNOW YOUR MUSCLES

Fill in the blank with the name of the muscles shown.

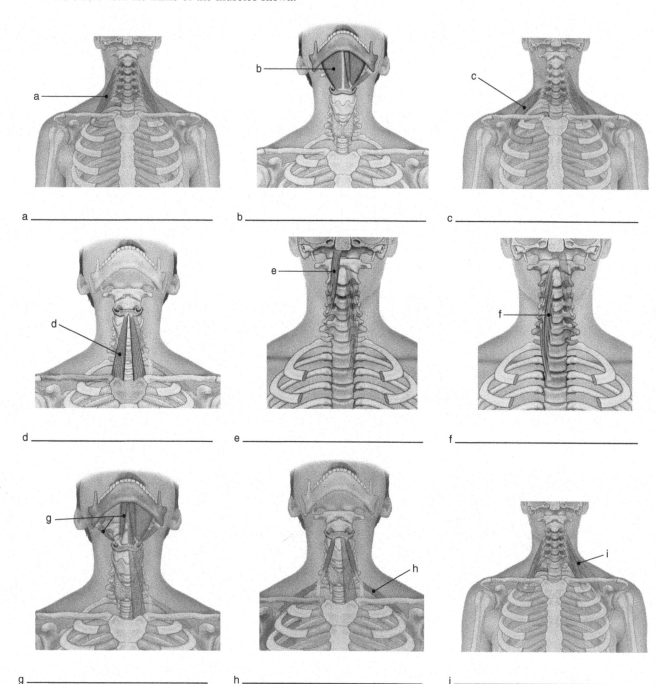

a _____

b _____

c _____

d _____

e _____

f _____

g _____

h _____

i _____

Score: ___/9

WHAT'S IN A NAME?

Match the muscle name from the right column to its meaning in the left column. Write your answer in the space provided. Each choice can be used only once.

Meaning

_____ 1. Straight muscle of the anterior head

_____ 2. Long muscle attaching to the head

_____ 3. Attaches to the hyoid and close to the molars

_____ 4. Attaches to the mandible and hyoid

_____ 5. Attaches to the styloid process and the hyoid

_____ 6. Long muscle of the neck

_____ 7. Attaches from the shoulder to the hyoid

_____ 8. Ladder-shaped muscle towards the back

_____ 9. Ladder-shaped muscle in the front

_____ 10. Attaches from the thyroid cartilage to the hyoid

_____ 11. Straight muscle of the lateral head

_____ 12. Attaches from the sternum to the thyroid cartilage

_____ 13. Attaches to the sternum and the hyoid

_____ 14. Ladder-shaped muscle in the middle

_____ 15. Muscle with two bellies

Muscle name

a. Sternohyoid

b. Thyrohyoid

c. Geniohyoid

d. Rectus capitis anterior

e. Posterior scalene

f. Omohyoid

g. Anterior scalene

h. Longus colli

i. Mylohyoid

j. Rectus capitis lateralis

k. Longus capitis

l. Middle scalene

m. Stylohyoid

n. Sternothyroid

o. Digastric

Score: ___/15

MATCHING ATTACHMENTS

Match each muscle from the word bank with its attachments. Write the answer in the column labeled *Muscle*. Each choice can be used only once.

Stylohyoid	Longus colli	Digastric
Sternothyroid	Longus capitis	Posterior scalene
Geniohyoid	Anterior scalene	Middle scalene
Mylohyoid	Rectus capitis anterior	Sternohyoid
Thyrohyoid	Rectus capitis lateralis	Omohyoid

Chapter **8** **Muscles of the Spine and Rib Cage**

Attachments	Muscle
1. Transverse processes of the cervical spine *to the* 1st rib	
2. Transverse processes of the cervical spine *to the* 1st rib	
3. Transverse processes of the cervical spine *to the* 2nd rib	
4. Temporal bone *to the* mandible	
5. Styloid process of the temporal bone *to the* hyoid	
6. Inner surface of the mandible *to the* hyoid	
7. Inner surface of the mandible *to the* hyoid	
8. Sternum *to the* hyoid	
9. Sternum *to the* thyroid cartilage	
10. Thyroid cartilage *to the* hyoid	
11. Scapula *to the* hyoid	
12. Anterior bodies and transverse processes of C3-T3 *to the* Anterior bodies and transverse processes of C2-C6 and the anterior arch of C1	
13. Transverse processes C3-C6 *to the* occiput	
14. The atlas (C1) *to the* occiput	
15. The atlas (C1) *to the* occiput	

Score: ___/15

Fill in the blanks with 1) the direction of movement, 2) the body part that is moving, and 3) the joint at which movement is occurring.

1. If a muscle crosses the spinal joints of the neck anteriorly with a vertical direction to its fibers, what action can it perform?

   _____ of the _____ at the _____ joint(s).

2. If a muscle crosses the spinal joints of the neck posteriorly with a vertical direction to its fibers, what action can it perform?

   _____ of the _____ at the _____ joint(s).

3. If a muscle crosses the spinal joints of the neck laterally on the left side with a vertical direction to its fibers, what action can it perform?

   _____ of the _____ at the _____ joint(s).

4. If a muscle attaches to the rib cage and its other attachment is superior to the rib cage attachment, what action can it perform?

   _____ of the _____ at the _____ joint(s).

5. If a muscle attaches to the rib cage and its other attachment is inferior to the rib cage attachment, what action can it perform?

   _____ of the _____ at the _____ joint(s).

6. If a muscle attaches to the mandible and its other attachment is inferior to the mandibular attachment, what action can it perform?

   _____ of the _____ at the _____ joint(s).

7. If a muscle attaches to the mandible and its other attachment is superior to the mandibular attachment, what action can it perform?

   _____ of the _____ at the _____ joint(s).

Score: ___/7

163

Place the corresponding joint action letter(s) in the blank(s) next to the muscle. The number of blanks next to each muscle name indicates the number of letters that should be placed next to that muscle.

Joint Action

a. Flexes the head

b. Laterally flexes the head

c. Flexes the neck

d. Flexes the head and neck

e. Laterally flexes the neck

f. Depresses the mandible

g. Elevates the hyoid bone

h. Depresses the hyoid bone and thyroid cartilage

i. Elevates the 1st rib

j. Elevates the 2nd rib

Muscle

1. Anterior scalene ____ ____ ____

2. Middle scalene ____ ____ ____

3. Posterior scalene ____ ____

4. Digastric ____ ____ ____

5. Stylohyoid ____

6. Geniohyoid ____ ____ ____

7. Mylohyoid ____ ____ ____

8. Infrahyoid muscles ____ ____

9. Longus colli ____

10. Longus capitis ____

11. Rectus capitis anterior ____

12. Rectus capitis lateralis ____

Score: ___/24

THE LONG AND THE SHORT OF IT – EXERCISE 1

For each joint action given, indicate whether the muscle shortens or lengthens.

1. Rectus capitis anterior: flexion of the head: _____

2. Mylohyoid: depression of the hyoid bone: _____

3. Posterior scalene: depression of the 2nd rib: _____

4. Longus capitis: extension of the head and neck: _____

5. Anterior scalene: elevation of the 1st rib: _____

Score: ___/5

THE LONG AND THE SHORT OF IT – EXERCISE 2

For each joint action given, fill in the blanks with a muscle that shortens and a muscle that lengthens. Please note that possible answers may be covered in another section.

1. Flexion of the neck:

   Shortens: _____ Lengthens: _____

2. Depression of the hyoid:

   Shortens: _____ Lengthens: _____

3. Elevation of the first rib:

   Shortens: _____ Lengthens: _____

4. Extension of the neck:

   Shortens: _____ Lengthens: _____

5. Elevates the hyoid:

   Shortens: _____ Lengthens: _____

Score: ___/10

MOVERS & ANTAGONISTS – EXERCISE 1

For each joint action stated, fill in the blank for a mover and antagonist of that joint action. Please choose your mover/antagonist pairs from the word bank below. Each pair can be used only once.

   Sternohyoid/Stylohyoid

   Digastric/Omohyoid

   Anterior scalene/Splenius capitis

   Right posterior scalene/Left posterior scalene

1. Right lateral flexion of the neck at the spinal joints:

   _____

2. Elevates the hyoid:

   _____

3. Flexes the neck at the spinal joints:

   _____

4. Depresses the hyoid:

   _____

Score: ___/4

165

For each joint action illustrated, the body part is being *slowly* moved in the direction indicated by the arrow. Circle whether the functional muscle group of the pair provided is contracting or relaxed. Then circle *how* the muscle group that is working is contracting (concentrically or eccentrically).

1.

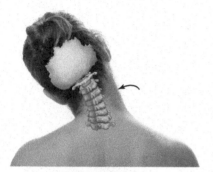

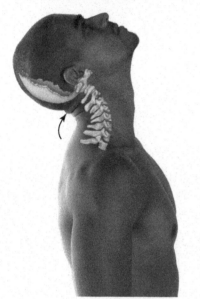

Movement:

Left lateral flexion of the neck at the spinal joints

Left lateral flexors: contracting/relaxed

Right lateral flexors: contracting/relaxed

What type of contraction is occurring?
concentric/eccentric

2.

Movement:

Flexion of the neck at the spinal joints

Flexors: contracting/relaxed

Extensors: contracting/relaxed

What type of contraction is occurring?
concentric/eccentric

3.

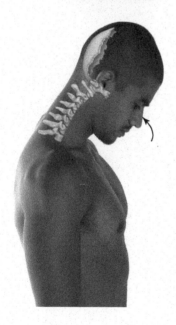

Movement:

Extension of the neck at the spinal joints

Extensors: contracting/relaxed

Flexors: contracting/relaxed

What type of contraction is occurring?
concentric/eccentric

Score: ___/12

MUSCLE STABILIZATIONS

Circle the letter of the best answer to the question.

1. Which of the following muscles can stabilize the cervical spinal joints and the head?
   a. Sternothyroid
   b. Middle scalene
   c. Thyrohyoid
   d. Rectus capitis anterior

2. Which of the following muscles can stabilize the 1st rib?
   a. Omohyoid
   b. Digastric
   c. Anterior scalene
   d. Posterior scalene

3. Which of the following muscles can stabilize the hyoid bone and the temporomandibular joints?
   a. Geniohyoid
   b. Posterior scalene
   c. Sternothyroid
   d. Rectus capitis lateralis

4. Which of the following muscles can stabilize the hyoid bone and the thyroid cartilage?
   a. Longus colli
   b. Mylohyoid
   c. Thyrohyoid
   d. Rectus capitis anterior

5. Which of the following muscles can stabilize the 2nd rib?
   a. Middle scalene
   b. Posterior scalene
   c. Mylohyoid
   d. Longus capitis

Score: ___/5

YOU'VE GOT NERVE!

Write the name of the corresponding innervation(s) from the list provided. Choices can be used more than once.

Cervical spinal nerves

Trigeminal nerve (CN V)

Facial nerve (CN VII)

Hypoglossal nerve (CN XII)

Cervical plexus

1. Anterior scalene _____

2. Middle scalene _____

3. Posterior scalene _____

4. Digastric _____

5. Stylohyoid _____

Chapter **8** **Muscles of the Spine and Rib Cage**

6. Geniohyoid _____

7. Mylohyoid _____

8. Sternohyoid _____

9. Sternothyroid _____

10. Thyrohyoid _____

11. Omohyoid _____

12. Longus colli _____

13. Longus capitis _____

14. Rectus capitis anterior _____

15. Rectus capitis lateralis _____

Score: ___/15

ARE YOU FEELING IT? – PALPATION

Fill in the blank with the best answer to the palpation question.

1. What muscle or muscle group is palpated immediately lateral to the sternocleidomastoid and immediately superior to

   the clavicle? _____

2. What muscle group is engaged and palpated immediately inferior to the mandible by asking the client to depress the mandible against gentle resistance?

   _____

3. What deep musculature is palpated immediately medial to the sternocleidomastoid?

   _____

4. When palpating the scalenes, how is the client asked to engage them?

   _____

Score: ___/4

CLINICALLY SPEAKING

Fill in the blank with the best answer for the treatment consideration question.

1. What muscles of the neck can be involved in thoracic outlet syndrome?

   _____

2. What muscles of the anterior neck can help to stabilize the temporomandibular joints?

   _____

3. What muscle is the prime mover of depression of the mandible?

_____

4. What blood vessel runs between the anterior and middle scalenes?

_____

Score: ___/4

MUSCLE MASH-UP

Fill in the blank with the best answer to the question.

1. What is the origin (proximal attachment) of the scalenes?

   _____

2. Where are the scalenes superficial? _____

3. Which ribs can the scalenes elevate? _____

4. Tight scalenes can cause what condition?

   _____

5. What likely occurs with pressure upon the carotid sinus?

   _____

6. What are the three muscles of the scalene group? _____

7. What are the four muscles of the suprahyoid group?

   _____

8. What are the names of the four muscles of the infrahyoid group?

   _____

9. Which infrahyoid muscle has two bellies? _____

10. Which deep muscle of the anterior neck and head runs from C6 to the occiput?

   _____

Score: ___/10

CROSSWORD PUZZLE

Use the clues to complete the crossword puzzle.

ACROSS

1 Largest scalene
4 Refers to the neck
6 The rectus capitis anterior is part of this group
7 Hyoid muscle in posterior triangle of neck
8 _____ scalene syndrome
11 Injury to neck muscles

DOWN

2 Located inferior to hyoid bone
3 Suprahyoid muscle with two heads
5 Deep to mylohyoid
8 Common attachment of rectus capitis anterior and lateralis
9 _____ outlet syndrome
10 Gastric means _____

Score: _/12

MINI CASE STUDIES

Fill in the blank with the best answer for the clinical case study questions.

1. What muscles of the anterior neck should be assessed in a client who presents with tingling into the upper extremity?

   _____

2. What anterior neck musculature should be assessed if a client complains of sore throat pain, especially when swallowing? _____

3. You are performing a neck assessment on a client who has recently added a lot of sit-ups to his exercise regime. What region of the neck should you pay particular attention to during the assessment? _____

4. A new client, who is a musician and plays the trumpet, presents with anterior neck pain. What muscle group should you assess? _____

Score: ___/4

MNEMONICS

Create your own mnemonic for the muscle group.

Erector spinae group:

Iliocostalis, Longissimus, Spinalis

I Love Spinach!

Now make one of your own:

I _____ L _____ S _____ .

Transversospinalis group:

Transversospinalis: Semispinalis, Multifidus, Rotatores

Try Smelling More Roses!

Now make one of your own:

T _____ S _____ M _____ R _____ .

Anterior abdominal wall muscles:

Transversus abdominis, Internal abdominal oblique, Rectus abdominis, External abdominal oblique

TIRE (think spare tire around the abdomen)

Now make one of your own:

T _____ I _____ R _____ E _____ .

Chapter **8** **Muscles of the Spine and Rib Cage**

Suprahyoid muscles:

Digastric, Stylohyoid, Mylohyoid, Geniohyoid

Don't Swallow My Gum!

Now make one of your own:

D _____ S _____ M _____ G _____ .

Infrahyoid muscles:

Sternohyoid, Sternothyroid, Thyrohyoid, Omohyoid

Super Sonic Take Off!

Now make one of your own:

S _____ S _____ T _____ O _____ .

Suboccipital muscles:

Rectus Capitis Posterior Major, Rectus Capitis Posterior Minor, Obliquus Capitis Superior, Obliquus Capitis Inferior

Roger Can Play Melodies; Roger Can Play Music; Oscar Can Swim; Oscar Can Ice skate!

Now make one of your own:

R _____ C _____ P _____ M _____

R _____ C _____ P _____ M _____

O _____ C _____ S _____

O _____ C _____ I _____

CHAPTERS 6–8 SUMMARY REVIEW - MULTIPLE CHOICE

Circle the letter of the best answer to the question.

1. What is the best method to discern the teres minor from the teres major when palpating?
   a. Teres minor will engage with lateral rotation.
   b. Teres major will engage with medial rotation.
   c. Both a and b
   d. None of the above

2. What muscle group is an extremely important stabilizer of the humeral head at the glenohumeral joint?
   a. Scalenes
   b. Erector spinae
   c. Rotator cuff (SITS)
   d. Pectoralis muscles

3. What is the name of the condition caused by compression of the ulnar nerve between the two heads of the flexor carpi ulnaris?
   a. Carpal tunnel syndrome
   b. Medial epicondylitis (golfer's elbow)
   c. Lateral epicondylitis (tennis elbow)
   d. Cubital tunnel syndrome

4. Which of the following is a TRUE statement?
   a. Abduction of the thumb is a sagittal plane motion.
   b. Flexion of the thumb is a frontal plane motion.
   c. Opposition of the thumb occurs when the thumb pad meets the pad of another finger.
   d. All of the above

5. Which muscle(s) is/are often involved in thoracic outlet syndrome?
   a. Erector spinae
   b. Scalenes
   c. Levator scapulae
   d. Rotator cuff (SITS)

9 Muscles of the Head

COLORING & LABELING

Use crayons or felt-tipped markers to color the muscles. Use the word banks to fill in the numbers that correspond to the names of the muscles, bones, and bony landmarks in the blanks provided.

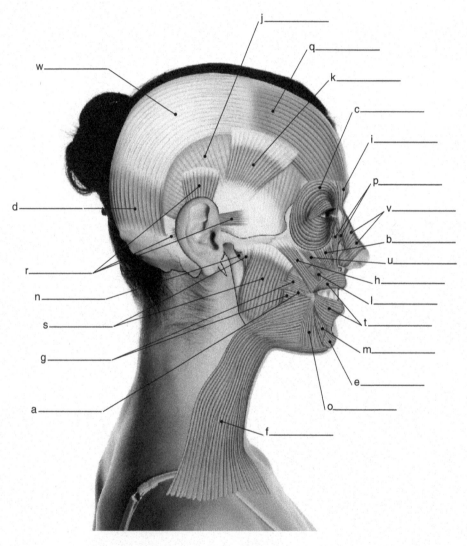

1. Auricularis muscles
2. Buccinator
3. Depressor anguli oris
4. Depressor labii inferioris
5. Frontalis of occipitofrontalis
6. Galea aponeurotica

7. Lateral pterygoid
8. Levator anguli oris
9. Levator labii superioris
10. Levator labii superioris alaeque nasi
11. Masseter

12. Mentalis
13. Nasalis
14. Occipitalis of occipitofrontalis
15. Orbicularis oculi
16. Orbicularis oris
17. Platysma

18. Procerus
19. Risorius
20. Temporalis (deep to fascia)
21. Temporoparietalis
22. Zygomaticus major
23. Zygomaticus minor

Score: ___/23

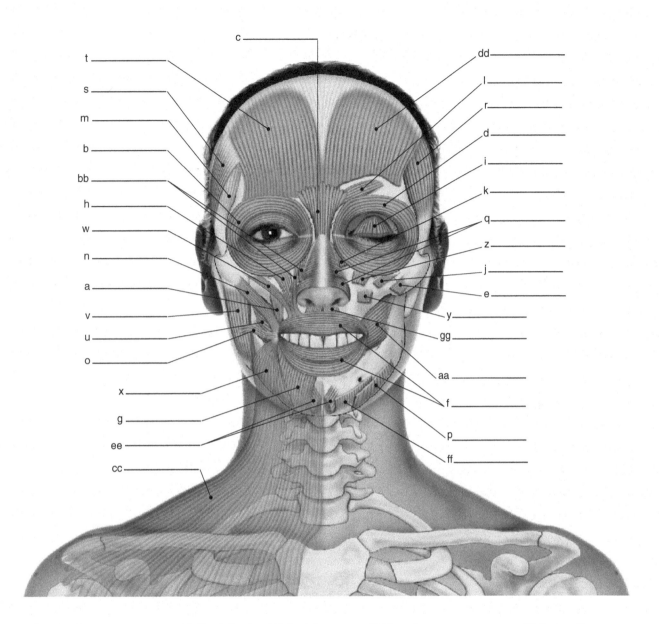

c ——————

t ——————

s ——————

m ——————

b ——————

bb ——————

h ——————

w ——————

n ——————

a ——————

v ——————

u ——————

o ——————

x ——————

g ——————

ee ——————

cc ——————

dd ——————

l ——————

r ——————

d ——————

i ——————

k ——————

q ——————

z ——————

j ——————

e ——————

y ——————

gg ——————

aa ——————

f ——————

p ——————

ff ——————

1. Buccinator

2. Buccinator

3. Corrugator supercilii

4. Depressor anguli oris

5. Depressor anguli oris (cut)

6. Depressor labii inferioris

7. Depressor labii inferioris (cut)

8. Depressor septi nasi

9. Frontalis (cut)

10. Frontalis of occipitofrontalis

11. Levator anguli oris

12. Levator anguli oris (cut)

13. Levator labii superioris

14. Levator labii superioris (cut)

15. Levator labii superioris alaeque nasi

16. Levator labii superioris alaeque nasi (cut)

17. Levator palpebrae superioris

18. Masseter

19. Mentalis

20. Nasalis

21. Orbicularis oculi

22. Orbicularis oculi (cut)

23. Orbicularis oris

24. Platysma

25. Procerus

26. Risorius

27. Temporalis

28. Temporalis

29. Temporoparietalis

30. Zygomaticus major

31. Zygomaticus major (cut)

32. Zygomaticus minor

33. Zygomaticus minor (cut)

Score: ___/33

175

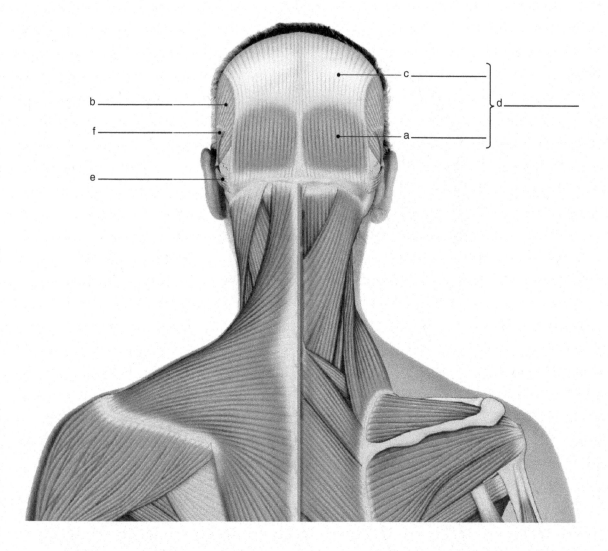

1. Auricularis posterior
2. Auricularis superior

3. Occipitalis
4. Occipitofrontalis

5. Galea aponeurotica
6. Temporalis (deep to fascia)

Score: ___/6

Section 1 tests your knowledge of muscles covered in pages 304–313 of the *Know the Body* textbook.

KNOW YOUR MUSCLES

Fill in the blank with the name of the muscles shown.

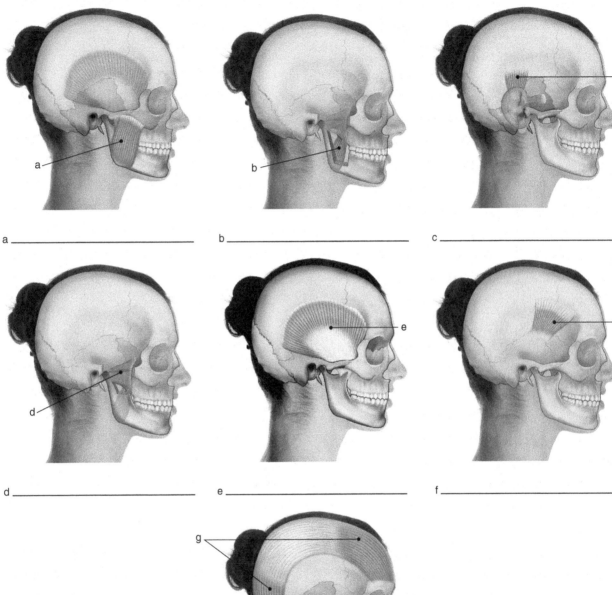

a _____

b _____

c _____

d _____

e _____

f _____

g _____

Score: ___/7

Match the muscle name from the right column to its meaning in the left column. Write your answer in the space provided. Each choice can be used only once.

Meaning

_____ 1. Muscle lying over the occipital and frontal bones

_____ 2. Muscle involved in chewing

_____ 3. Muscle behind to the ear

_____ 4. Muscle attaching to the temporal bone

_____ 5. Muscle attaching to the sphenoid bone more laterally than another muscle

_____ 6. Muscle attaching to the sphenoid bone more medially than another muscle

_____ 7. Muscle lying over the temporal and parietal bones

_____ 8. Muscle in front of the ear

_____ 9. Muscle above to the ear

Muscle name

a. Temporalis

b. Masseter

c. Lateral pterygoid

d. Medial pterygoid

e. Auricularis anterior

f. Auricularis superior

g. Auricularis posterior

h. Occipitofrontalis

i. Temporoparietalis

Score: ___/9

MATCHING ATTACHMENTS

Match the muscle from the word bank with its attachments. Write the answer in the column labeled *Muscle*. Each choice can be used only once.

Auricularis posterior	Lateral pterygoid	Masseter
Auricularis anterior	Medial pterygoid	Temporalis
Auricularis superior	Temporoparietalis	Occipitofrontalis

Attachments	**Muscle**
1. Temporal fossa *to the* coronoid process of the ramus of the mandible	
2. Inferior margins of both the zygomatic bone and the zygomatic arch of the temporal bone *to the* angle, ramus, and coronoid process of the mandible	
3. Sphenoid bone *to the* mandible and temporomandibular joint capsule	
4. Sphenoid bone *to the* internal surface of the mandible	

5. Galea aponeurotica *to the* anterior ear	
6. Galea aponeurotica *to the* superior ear	
7. Temporal bone *to the* posterior ear	
8. Occipital bone and the temporal bone *to the* fascia and skin overlying the frontal bone	
9. Lateral border of the galea aponeurotica *to the* fascia superior to the ear	

Score: ___/9

THE BIG PICTURE – FUNCTIONAL GROUPS

Fill in the blanks with 1) the direction of movement, 2) the body part that is moving, and 3) the joint(s) at which movement is occurring.

1. If a muscle attaches to the mandible and its other attachment is inferior to the mandibular attachment, what action can it perform?

   _____ of the _____ at the _____ joint(s).

2. If a muscle attaches to the mandible and its other attachment is superior to the mandibular attachment, what action can it perform?

   _____ of the _____ at the _____ joint(s).

3. If a muscle attaches to the mandible and its other attachment is medial to the mandibular attachment, what action can it perform?

   _____ of the _____ at the _____ joint(s).

4. If a muscle attaches to the mandible and its other attachment is anterior to the mandibular attachment, what action can it perform?

   _____ of the _____ at the _____ joint(s).

5. If a muscle attaches to the mandible and its other attachment is posterior to the mandibular attachment, what action can it perform?

   _____ of the _____ at the _____ joint(s).

Score: ___/5

179

MATCHING ACTIONS

Place the corresponding joint action letter(s) in the blank(s) next to the muscle. The number of blanks next to each muscle name indicates the number of letters that should be placed next to that muscle. Choices can be used more than once.

Joint Action

a. Elevates the mandible

b. Protracts the mandible

c. Contralaterally deviates the mandible

d. Posteriorly draws the scalp

e. Anteriorly draws the ear

f. Elevates the ear

g. Posteriorly draws the ear

Muscle

1. Temporalis ____

2. Masseter ____

3. Lateral pterygoid ____ ____

4. Medial pterygoid ____ ____ ____

5. Auricularis anterior ____

6. Auricularis superior ____

7. Auricularis posterior ____

8. Occipitofrontalis ____

9. Temporoparietalis ____

Score: ___/12

THE LONG AND THE SHORT OF IT – EXERCISE 1

For each joint action given, indicate whether the muscle shortens or lengthens.

1. Temporalis: elevation of the mandible: _____

2. Masseter: depression of the mandible: _____

3. Lateral pterygoid: ipsilateral deviation of the mandible: _____

4. Occipitofrontalis: drawing of the scalp posteriorly: _____

5. Auricularis posterior: drawing of the ear posteriorly: _____

Score: ___/5

THE LONG AND THE SHORT OF IT – EXERCISE 2

For each joint action given, fill in the blanks with a muscle that shortens and a muscle that lengthens. Please note that possible answers may be covered in another section.

1. Elevation of the mandible:

   Shortens: _____   Lengthens: _____

2. Depression of the mandible:

   Shortens: _____   Lengthens: _____

3. Drawing of the ear anteriorly:

   Shortens: _____   Lengthens: _____

Chapter **9** **Muscles of the Head**

4. Drawing of the ear posteriorly:

   Shortens: _____   Lengthens: _____

5. Contralateral deviation of the mandible:

   Shortens: _____

MOVERS & ANTAGONISTS – EXERCISE 1

For each joint action stated, fill in the blank for a mover and antagonist of that joint action. Please choose your mover/antagonist pairs from the word bank below. Each pair can be used once and only once.

   Temporalis/Digastric

   Right lateral pterygoid/Left medial pterygoid

1. Elevates the mandible at the temporomandibular joints:

   _____

2. Left lateral deviation of the mandible at the temporomandibular joints:

   _____

For each joint action illustrated, the body part is being *slowly* moved in the direction indicated by the arrow. Circle whether the functional muscle group of the pair provided is contracting or relaxed. Then circle *how* the muscle group that is working is contracting (concentrically or eccentrically).

1.

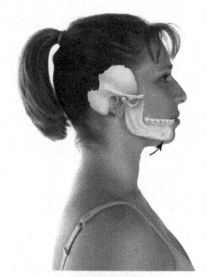

Movement:

Elevation of the mandible at the temporomandibular joints

Elevators: contracting/relaxed

Depressors: contracting/relaxed

What type of contraction is occurring?
concentric/eccentric

2.

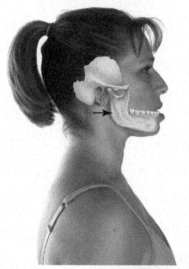

Movement:

Protraction of the mandible at the temporomandibular joints

Protractors: contracting/relaxed

Retractors: contracting/relaxed

What type of contraction is occurring?
concentric/eccentric

3.

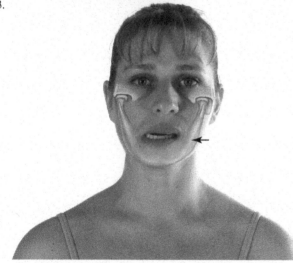

Movement:

Right lateral deviation of the mandible at the temporomandibular joints

Right lateral deviators: contracting/relaxed

Left lateral deviators: contracting/relaxed

What type of contraction is occurring?
concentric/eccentric

Score: ___/9

MUSCLE STABILIZATIONS

Circle the letter of the best answer to the question.

1. Which of the following muscles can stabilize the mandible at the temporomandibular joints?
   a. Auricularis superior
   b. Auricularis posterior
   c. Occipitofrontalis
   d. Medial pterygoid

2. Which of the following muscles can stabilize the mandible at the temporomandibular joints?
   a. Temporoparietalis
   b. Masseter
   c. Auricularis anterior
   d. Occipitofrontalis

Score: ___/2

YOU'VE GOT NERVE!

Write the name of the corresponding innervation from the list provided. Choices will be used more than once.

Trigeminal nerve (CN V)

Facial nerve (CN VII)

1. Temporalis _____

2. Masseter _____

3. Lateral pterygoid _____

4. Medial pterygoid _____

5. Auricularis anterior _____

6. Auricularis superior _____

7. Auricularis posterior _____

8. Occipitofrontalis _____

9. Temporoparietalis _____

Score: ___/9

ARE YOU FEELING IT? – PALPATION

Fill in the blank with the best answer to the palpation question.

1. What muscle is palpated superior to the ear as the client alternately clenches the teeth and relaxes the jaw?

   _____

2. What muscle is palpated inside the mouth by going along the external surfaces of the upper teeth and then palpating posteriorly and superiorly? _____

3. What do we ask the client to do to engage and palpate the masseter?

_____

4. What do we ask the client to do to engage and palpate the occipitofrontalis?

_____

Score: ___/4

CLINICALLY SPEAKING

Fill in the blank with the best answer for the treatment consideration question.

1. What is the relationship between the direction of fibers of the masseter and medial pterygoid?

_____

2. What muscle of mastication has a thick layer of fascia that overlies it?

_____

3. What facial muscle has fibers that attach into the capsule of the temporomandibular joint?

_____

4. What muscle is often stated to be the most powerful muscle in the human body, proportional to its size?

_____

5. What muscle group of the head is highly developed in many animals, but often non-functional in humans?

_____

Score: ___/5

MUSCLE MASH-UP

Fill in the blank with the best answer to the question.

1. What muscle of the scalp can create a facial expression of surprise or shock?

_____

2. What are the names of the four major muscles of mastication?

_____

3. Which is deeper, the masseter or medial pterygoid?

_____

4. Which two muscles are palpated from inside the mouth?

_____

5. What are the two bellies of the occipitofrontalis? _____

6. Where is the masseter palpated?

   _____

7. What are the two common actions of the medial and lateral pterygoids?

   _____

8. What muscle is palpated by following the internal surface of the lower teeth?

   _____

9. Name the three auricularis muscles.

   _____

10. What structure separates the two bellies of the occipitofrontalis?

    _____

Score: ___/10

MINI CASE STUDIES

Fill in the blank with the best answer for the clinical case study questions.

1. A client comes to you and states that she has damage to the articular disc of her temporomandibular joint. What muscle do you suspect most likely contributes to this condition?

   _____

2. A client presents and states that he has temporomandibular joint syndrome. Which four muscles are the most important for you to assess?

   _____

3. A client experiences chronic tension headaches. Treatment to what scalp muscle most likely helps?

   _____

4. A client presents with pain in the cheek area that is exacerbated when biting down hard. What muscle should be assessed?

   _____

Score: ___/4

Use the clues to complete the crossword puzzle.

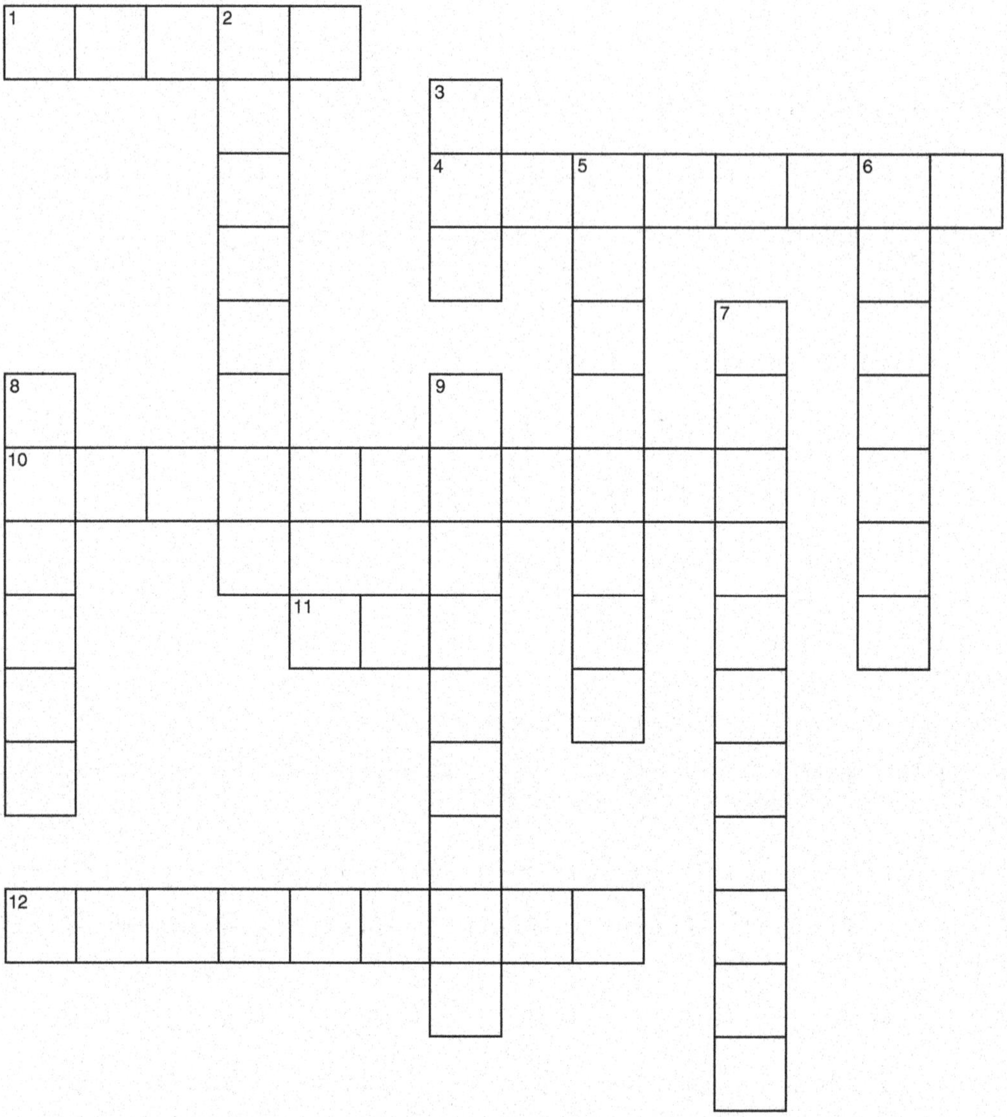

ACROSS

1 Temporal landmark that is deeper in carnivores
4 Attaches externally to the angle of the mandible
10 Moves the ears
11 Innervates the major muscles of mastication (acronym of 2 words)
12 Wing-shaped

DOWN

2 Origin of both pterygoids
3 Temporomandibular joint (acronym)
5 Higher than
6 The lateral pterygoid does not _____ the mandible at the temporomandibular joints
7 Chewing
8 Nerve that innervates the facial muscles
9 Action of the masseter and medial pterygoid

Score: ___/12

Section 2 tests your knowledge of muscles covered in pages 314–334 of the *Know the Body* textbook.

KNOW YOUR MUSCLES

Fill in the blank with the name of the muscles shown.

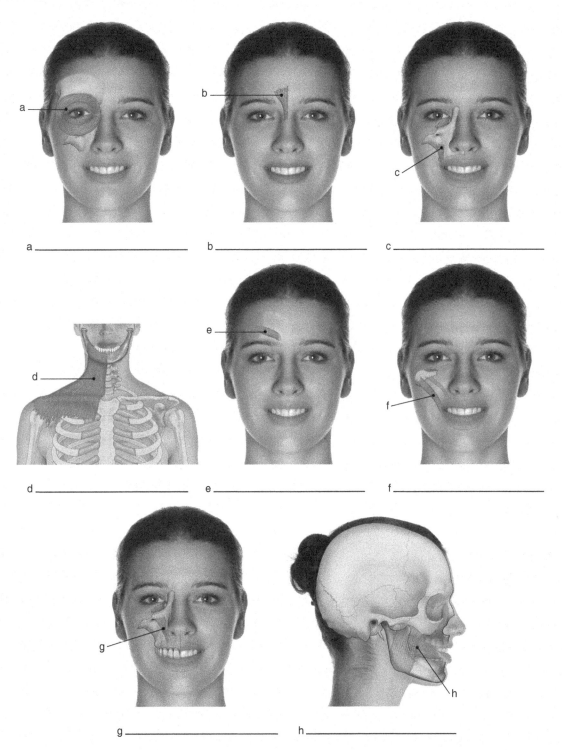

a _____

b _____

c _____

d _____

e _____

f _____

g _____

h _____

Score: ___/8

187

Match the muscle name from the right column to its meaning in the left column. Write your answer in the space provided. Each choice can be used only once.

Meaning

_____ 1. Muscle that depresses the angle of the mouth

_____ 2. Muscle that elevates the angle of the mouth

_____ 3. Muscle found in the cheek region

_____ 4. Muscle that elevates the upper lip

_____ 5. Muscle that encircles the eye

_____ 6. Muscle that elevates the upper eyelid

_____ 7. A smaller muscle attaching to the zygomatic bone

_____ 8. Muscle that is related to the chin

_____ 9. Muscle that depresses the nasal septum

_____ 10. Muscle involved with the nose

_____ 11. Muscle that wrinkles the skin of the eyebrow

_____ 12. Muscle that elevates the upper lip and is involved with the ala of the nose

_____ 13. A larger muscle attaching to the zygomatic bone

_____ 14. Muscle that is broad and flat

_____ 15. Muscle that depresses the lower lip

_____ 16. Helps create the expression of superiority of a nobleman or prince

_____ 17. Muscle that encircles the mouth

_____ 18. Muscle involved with laughing

Muscle name

a. Levator palpebrae superioris

b. Zygomaticus major

c. Procerus

d. Levator anguli oris

e. Levator labii superioris

f. Buccinator

g. Depressor labii inferioris

h. Depressor septi nasi

i. Mentalis

j. Depressor anguli oris

k. Orbicularis oculi

l. Risorius

m. Orbicularis oris

n. Corrugator supercilii

o. Nasalis

p. Levator labii superioris alaeque nasi

q. Zygomaticus minor

r. Platysma

Score: ___/18

Match each muscle from the word bank with its attachments. Write the answer in the column labeled *Muscle*. Each choice will be used only once.

Levator labii superioris alaeque nasi	Depressor labii inferioris
Levator anguli oris	Depressor septi nasi
Levator palpebrae superioris	Depressor anguli oris
Levator labii superioris	Corrugator supercilii
Zygomaticus major	Zygomaticus minor
Orbicularis oculi	Orbicularis oris
Buccinator	Platysma
Procerus	Risorius
Mentalis	Nasalis

Attachments	Muscle
1. Encircles the eye (from the medial side of the eye, it returns to the medial side of the eye)	
2. Sphenoid bone *to the* upper eyelid	
3. Inferior frontal bone *to the* fascia and skin deep to the eyebrow	
4. Fascia and skin medial to the eyebrow *to the* fascia and skin over the nasal bone	
5. Maxilla *to the* cartilage of the nose and the opposite-side nasalis muscle	
6. Maxilla *to the* cartilage of the nose	
7. Maxilla *to the* Upper lip and the nose	
8. Maxilla *to the* Upper lip	
9. Zygomatic bone *to the* upper lip	
10. Zygomatic bone *to the* angle of the mouth	
11. Maxilla *to the* angle of the mouth	

12. Fascia and skin superficial to the masseter *to the* angle of the mouth	
13. Maxilla and the mandible *to the* lips	
14. Mandible *to the* Angle of the mouth	
15. Mandible *to the* lower lip	
16. Mandible *to the* fascia and skin of the chin	
17. Surrounds the mouth	
18. Subcutaneous fascia of the superior chest *to the* mandible and the subcutaneous fascia of the lower face	

Score: ___/18

THE BIG PICTURE – FUNCTIONAL GROUPS

Fill in the blank with the best answer to the question.

1. If a muscle attaches to the angle of the mouth and its other attachment is superior to that attachment, which way will

   it move the angle of the mouth? _____

2. If a muscle attaches to the angle of the mouth and its other attachment is inferior to that attachment, which way will

   it move the angle of the mouth? _____

3. If a muscle attaches to the angle of the mouth and its other attachment is lateral to that attachment, which way will it
   move the angle of the mouth?

   _____

4. If a muscle attaches to the upper lip and its other attachment is superior to that attachment, which way will it move

   the upper lip? _____

5. If a muscle attaches to the lower lip and its other attachment is inferior to that attachment, which way will it move the

   lower lip? _____

Score: ___/5

MATCHING ACTIONS

Place the corresponding joint action letter(s) in the blank(s) next to the muscle. The number of blanks next to each muscle name indicates the number of letters that should be placed next to that muscle.

Joint Action

a. Closing and squinting of the eye

b. Elevates the upper eyelid

c. Inferomedially draws the eyebrow

d. Draws the medial eyebrow down

e. Wrinkles the skin of the nose upward

f. Constricts the nostril

g. Flares the nostril

h. Elevates the upper lip

i. Elevates the lower lip

j. Depresses the lower lip

k. Everts the lower lip

l. Protracts the lower lip

m. Protracts the lips

n. Elevates the angle of the mouth

o. Depresses the angle of the mouth

p. Laterally draws the angle of the mouth

q. Compresses the cheek against the teeth

r. Closes the mouth

s. Draws up the skin of the superior chest and neck

Muscle

1. Orbicularis oculi ____

2. Levator palpebrae superioris ____

3. Corrugator supercilii ____

4. Procerus ____ ____

5. Nasalis ____ ____

6. Depressor septi nasi ____

7. Levator labii superioris alaeque nasi ____ ____

8. Levator labii superioris ____

9. Zygomaticus minor ____

10. Zygomaticus major ____

11. Levator anguli oris ____

12. Risorius ____

13. Buccinator ____

14. Depressor anguli oris ____

15. Depressor labii inferioris ____

16. Mentalis ____ ____ ____

17. Orbicularis oris ____ ____

18. Platysma ____

Score: ___/24

THE LONG AND THE SHORT OF IT – EXERCISE 1

For each joint action given, indicate whether the muscle shortens or lengthens.

1. Orbicularis oculi: opening of the eye: _____

2. Zygomaticus minor: elevation of the upper lip: _____

3. Orbicularis oris: opening of the mouth: _____

4. Mentalis: eversion of the lower lip: _____

5. Corrugator supercilii: drawing of the eyebrow superolaterally: _____

Score: ___/5

Chapter **9** **Muscles of the Head**

THE LONG AND THE SHORT OF IT – EXERCISE 2

For each joint action given, fill in the blanks with a muscle that shortens and a muscle that lengthens. Please note that possible answers may be covered in another section.

1. Constriction of the nostril:

    Shortens: _____   Lengthens: _____

2. Elevation of the angle of the mouth:

    Shortens: _____   Lengthens: _____

3. Elevation of the lower lip:

    Shortens: _____   Lengthens: _____

4. Depression of the angle of the mouth:

    Shortens: _____   Lengthens: _____

5. Flaring of the nostril:

    Shortens: _____   Lengthens: _____

Score: ___/10

MOVERS & ANTAGONISTS – EXERCISE 1

For each joint action stated, fill in the blank for a mover and antagonist of that joint action. Please choose your mover/antagonist pairs from the word bank below. Each pair can be used only once.

    Auricularis anterior/Auricularis posterior

    Levator anguli oris/Depressor anguli oris

    Nasalis/Depressor septi nasi

    Occipitofrontalis/Procerus

1. Elevates the eyebrow: _____

2. Draws the ear anteriorly: _____

3. Flares the nostril: _____

4. Elevates the angle of the mouth: _____

Score: ___/4

Write the name of the corresponding innervation from the list provided. Choices will be used more than once.

Facial nerve (CN VII)

Oculomotor nerve (CN III)

1. Orbicularis oculi _____

2. Levator palpebrae superioris _____

3. Corrugator supercilii _____

4. Procerus _____

5. Nasalis _____

6. Depressor septi nasi _____

7. Levator labii superioris alaeque nasi _____

8. Levator labii superioris _____

9. Zygomaticus minor _____

10. Zygomaticus major _____

11. Levator anguli oris _____

12. Risorius _____

13. Buccinator _____

14. Depressor anguli oris _____

15. Depressor labii inferioris _____

16. Mentalis _____

17. Orbicularis oris _____

18. Platysma _____

Score: ___/18

Fill in the blank with the best answer to the palpation question.

1. To palpate the orbicularis oculi, what do we ask the client to do?

_____

2. What muscle is palpated at the medial eyebrow when the client frowns?

_____

3. What muscle is palpated over the bridge of the nose as the client wrinkles the skin of the nose upward?

_____

4. What muscle is palpated in the cheeks as the client forcefully expels air from the mouth?

_____

5. To palpate the platysma, what do we ask the client to do?

_____

Score: ___/5

CLINICALLY SPEAKING

Fill in the blank with the best answer to the treatment consideration question.

1. The chronic contraction of what muscle causes crow's-feet?

_____

2. Explain the effects of botox on the facial musculature.

_____

3. The contraction of what muscles creates the Dracula expression?

_____

4. The contraction of what muscle is reminiscent of the Creature from the Black Lagoon?

_____

5. These muscles are involved when blowing up a balloon.

_____

6. What muscle of facial expression is useful when drinking a beverage?

_____

Score: ___/6

MUSCLE MASH-UP

Fill in the blank with the best answer to the question.

1. What muscle creates an expression of disdain or superiority?

_____

2. Which two muscles of facial expression attach to the zygomatic bone?

_____

3. Which facial muscle has the longest name?

_____

4. What are the names of the three muscles of facial expression of the eye?

_____

5. Name the three muscles of the nose involved in facial expression.

_____

6. What muscle is a muscle of expression for both the nose and mouth?

_____

7. What muscle attaches from the maxilla and mandible to the lips?

_____

8. What cranial nerve innervates almost every muscle of facial expression?

_____

9. What muscle is used to wink?

_____

10. Bringing the medial eyebrows down can help to shield the eyes from what?

_____

Score: ___/10

CROSSWORD PUZZLE

Use the clues to complete the crossword puzzle.

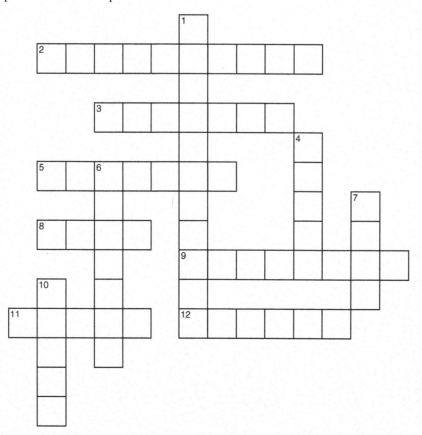

ACROSS

2 Depressor septi nasi _____ the nostril
3 Origin (superior attachment) of levator anguli oris
5 Another name for the levator anguli oris
8 Refers to the nose
9 Laughing
11 Refers to the lip
12 Depressor labii inferioris creates a look of _____

DOWN

1 Surrounds
4 Zygomaticus muscle to the angle of the mouth
6 Flares the nostril
7 With the mentalis, you can_____
10 Larger

Score: ___/12

MINI CASE STUDIES

Fill in the blank with the best answer for the clinical case study questions.

1. What muscle is most likely tightened in a person who squints a lot?

_____

2. What muscle is greatly strengthened in a professional musician who plays a brass instrument?

_____

3. What muscle is strengthened in a person who whistles often?

_____

4. What is likely true about a person who has many facial wrinkles?

_____

Score: ___/4

MNEMONICS

Create your own mnemonic for the muscle group.

Major muscles of mastication:

<u>T</u>emporalis, <u>M</u>asseter, <u>M</u>edial <u>P</u>terygoid, <u>L</u>ateral <u>P</u>terygoid

<u>T</u>iny <u>M</u>ice <u>M</u>ake <u>P</u>retty <u>L</u>ittle <u>P</u>aw prints!

Now make one of your own:

T _____ M _____ M _____ P _____ L _____ P _____

Muscles of the scalp:

<u>O</u>ccipitofrontalis, <u>T</u>emporoparietalis, <u>A</u>uricularis <u>M</u>uscles

<u>O</u>ld <u>T</u>oupees <u>A</u>lways <u>M</u>ove!

Now make one of your own:

O _____ T _____ A _____ M _____.

Facial expression muscles of the nose:

<u>P</u>rocerus, <u>N</u>asalis, <u>D</u>epressor <u>S</u>epti <u>N</u>asi

<u>P</u>ink <u>N</u>oses <u>D</u>o <u>S</u>weetly <u>N</u>uzzle!

Now make one of your own:

P _____ N _____ D _____ S _____ N _____.

Facial expression muscles of the eye:

<u>O</u>rbicularis <u>O</u>culi, <u>L</u>evator <u>P</u>alpebrae <u>S</u>uperioris, <u>C</u>orrugator <u>S</u>upercilii

<u>O</u>nly <u>O</u>ne <u>L</u>olli <u>P</u>op <u>S</u>tarts <u>C</u>hildren <u>S</u>ucking!

Now make one of your own:

O _____ O _____ L _____ P _____ S _____ C _____

S _____.

Use crayons or felt-tipped markers to color the muscles. Use the word banks to fill in the numbers that correspond to the names of the muscles in the blanks provided.

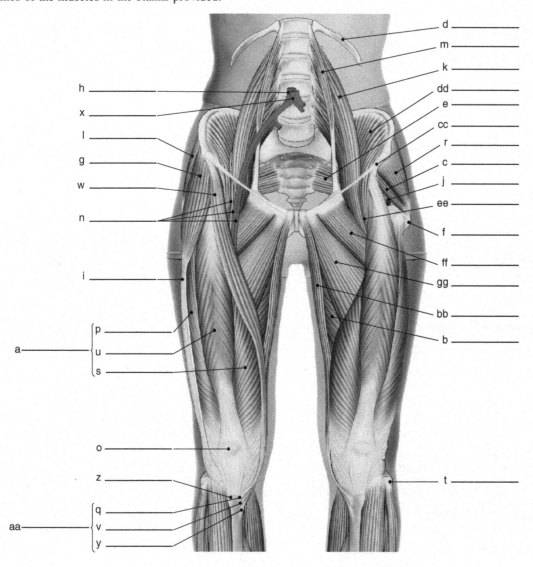

1. 12th rib	10. Gracilis	18. Patella	26. Rectus femoris
2. Abdominal aorta	11. Greater trochanter of femur	19 Pectineus	27. Sartorius
3. Adductor longus	12. Head of fibula	20. Pes anserine tendon	28. Sartorius
4. Adductor magnus	13. Iliacus	21. Piriformis	29. Semitendinosus
5. Femoral nerve, artery, and vein	14. Iliopsoas	22. Piriformis	30. Tensor fasciae latae
6. Gluteus medius	15. Iliotibial band	23. Psoas major	31. Tibial tuberosity
7. Gluteus medius	16. Inferior vena cava	24. Psoas minor	32. Vastus lateralis
8. Gluteus minimus	17. Inguinal ligament	25. Quadriceps femoris	33. Vastus medialis
9. Gracilis			

Score: ___/33

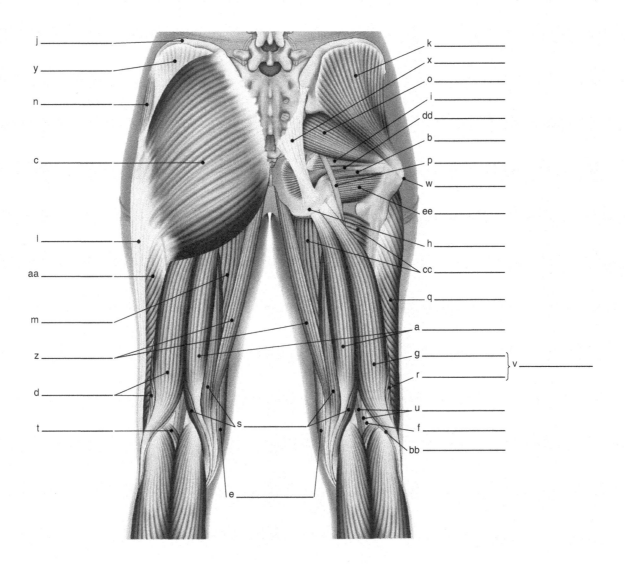

j _____

y _____

n _____

c _____

l _____

aa _____

m _____

z _____

d _____

t _____

e _____

k _____

x _____

o _____

i _____

dd _____

b _____

p _____

w _____

ee _____

h _____

cc _____

q _____

a _____

g _____

r _____

} v _____

u _____

f _____

bb _____

s _____

1. Adductor magnus	9. Gracilis	17. Piriformis	25. Semitendinosus
2. Adductor magnus	10. Greater trochanter of femur	18. Plantaris	26. Short head
3. Biceps femoris	11. Iliac crest	19. Popliteal artery and vein	27. Superior gemellus
4. Biceps femoris	12. Iliotibial band	20. Quadratus femoris	28. Tensor fasciae latae
5. Common fibular nerve	13. Inferior gemellus	21. Sacrotuberous ligament	29. Tibial nerve
6. Gluteus maximus	14. Ischial tuberosity	22. Sartorius	30. Vastus lateralis
7. Gluteus medius	15. Long head	23. Sciatic nerve	31. Vastus lateralis
8. Gluteus medius (deep to fascia)	16. Obturator internus	24. Semimembranosus	

Score: ___/31

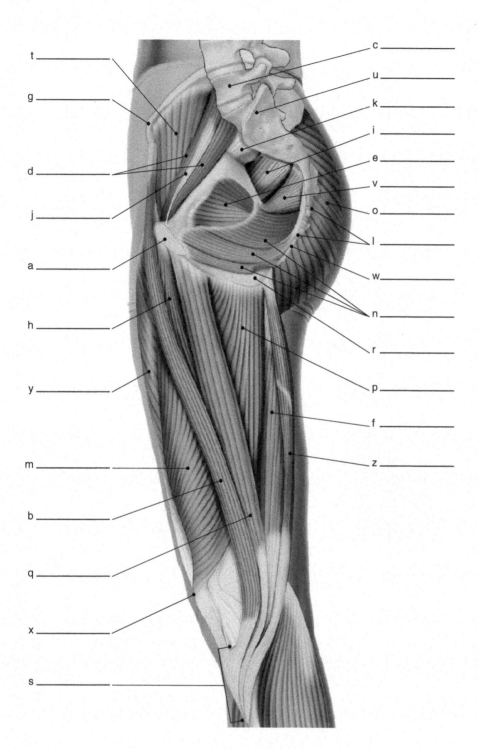

t _____   c _____

g _____   u _____

    k _____

    i _____

d _____   e _____

    v _____

j _____   o _____

    l _____

a _____

    w _____

h _____

    n _____

    r _____

y _____

    p _____

    f _____

m _____

    z _____

b _____

q _____

x _____

s _____

1. Adductor longus	8. Gluteus maximus	15. Patella	21. Rectus femoris
2. Adductor magnus	9. Gracilis	16. Pes anserine tendon	22. Sacrum
3. Anococcygeal ligament	10. Iliacus	17. Piriformis	23. Sartorius
4. Anterior sacroiliac ligaments	11. Ischial tuberosity	18. Psoas major	24. Semimembranosus
5. Anterior superior iliac spine	12. L5	19. Psoas minor	25. Semitendinosus
6. Coccygeus	13. Levator ani	20. Pubic symphysis	26. Vastus medialis
7. Coccyx	14. Obturator internus		

Score: ___/26

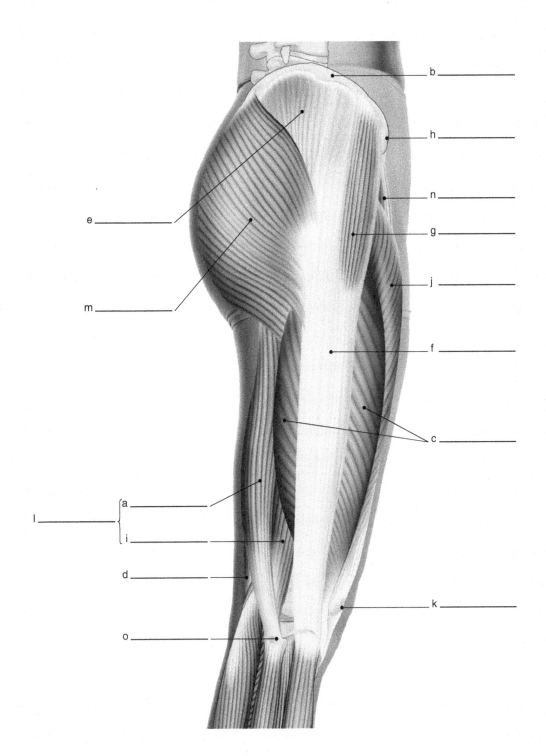

b _____

h _____

n _____

g _____

j _____

f _____

c _____

e _____

m _____

l _____
a _____
i _____

d _____

k _____

o _____

1. Anterior superior iliac spine
2. Biceps femoris
3. Gluteus maximus
4. Gluteus medius (deep to fascia)
5. Head of fibula

6. Iliac crest
7. Iliotibial band
8. Long head
9. Patella
10. Rectus femoris

11. Sartorius
12. Semimembranosus
13. Short head
14. Tensor fasciae latae
15. Vastus lateralis

Score: ___/15

Chapter **10** **Muscles of the Pelvis and Thigh**

Section 1 tests your knowledge of the muscles covered in pages 346–354 of the *Know the Body* textbook.

KNOW YOUR MUSCLES

Fill in the blank with the name of the muscles shown.

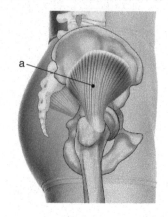

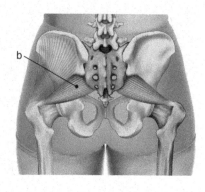

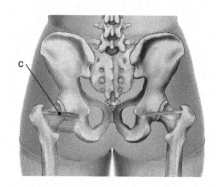

a _____

b _____

c _____

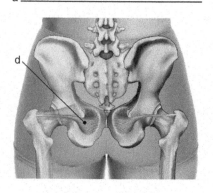

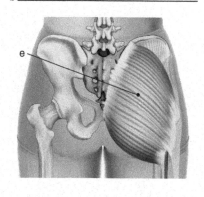

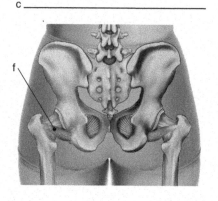

d _____

e _____

f _____

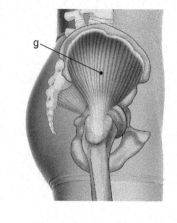

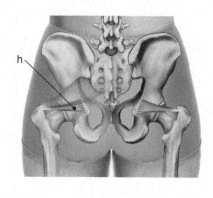

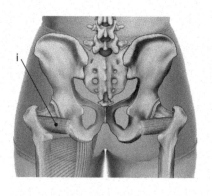

g _____

h _____

i _____

Score: ___/9

WHAT'S IN A NAME?

Match the muscle name from the right column to its meaning in the left column. Write your answer in the space provided. Each choice will be used only once.

Meaning

_____ 1. Muscle attaches to the internal surface of the obturator foramen

_____ 2. Muscle attaches to the external surface of the obturator foramen

_____ 3. Smallest muscle of the buttock region

_____ 4. Medium-sized muscle of the buttock region

_____ 5. Is the more inferior muscle of a pair of similar muscles

_____ 6. Is the more superior muscle of a pair of similar muscles

_____ 7. Square-shaped muscle attaching to the femur

_____ 8. Largest muscle of the buttock region

_____ 9. Pear-shaped muscle

Muscle name

a. Gluteus maximus

b. Quadratus femoris

c. Superior gemellus

d. Inferior gemellus

e. Gluteus minimus

f. Obturator externus

g. Gluteus medius

h. Obturator internus

i. Piriformis

Score: ___/9

MATCHING ATTACHMENTS

Match each muscle from the word bank with its attachments. Write the answer in the column labeled *Muscle*. Each choice will be used only once.

Superior gemellus   Gluteus maximus   Piriformis

Inferior gemellus   Gluteus medius   Obturator internus

Quadratus femoris   Gluteus minimus   Obturator externus

Attachments	Muscle
1. Posterior iliac crest, the posterolateral sacrum, and the coccyx *to the* Iliotibial band (ITB) and the gluteal tuberosity of the femur	
2. External ilium *to the* greater trochanter of the femur	
3. External ilium *to the* greater trochanter of the femur	
4. Anterior sacrum *to the* greater trochanter of the femur	
5. Ischial spine *to the* greater trochanter of the femur	

203

6. Internal surface of the pelvic bone surrounding the obturator foramen *to the* Greater trochanter of the femur	
7. Ischial tuberosity *to the* Greater trochanter of the femur	
8. External surface of the pelvic bone surrounding the obturator foramen *to the* Trochanteric fossa of the femur	
9. Ischial tuberosity *to the* intertrochanteric crest of the femur	

Score: ___/9

THE BIG PICTURE – FUNCTIONAL GROUPS

Fill in the blanks with 1) the direction of movement, 2) the body part that is moving, and 3) the joint at which movement is occurring.

1. If a muscle crosses the hip joint anteriorly with a vertical direction to its fibers, what two actions can it perform?

_____ of the _____ at the _____ joint(s).

_____ of the _____ at the _____ joint(s).

2. If a muscle crosses the hip joint posteriorly with a vertical direction to its fibers, what two actions can it perform?

_____ of the _____ at the _____ joint(s).

_____ of the _____ at the _____ joint(s).

3. If a muscle crosses the hip joint laterally with a vertical direction to its fibers, what action can it perform?

_____ of the _____ at the _____ joint(s).

4. If a muscle crosses the hip joint medially with a vertical direction to its fibers, what action can it perform?

_____ of the _____ at the _____ joint(s).

5. What is the reverse action of extension of the thigh at the hip joint?

_____ of the _____ at the _____ joint(s).

6. What is the reverse action of lateral rotation of the thigh at the hip joint?

_____ of the _____ at the _____ joint(s).

Score: ___/6

Chapter **10** **Muscles of the Pelvis and Thigh**

MATCHING ACTIONS

Place the corresponding joint action letter(s) in the blank(s) next to the muscle. The number of blanks next to each muscle name indicates the number of letters that should be placed next to that muscle.

Joint Actions

a. Flexes the thigh at the hip joint

b. Extends the thigh at the hip joint

c. Horizontally extends the thigh at the hip joint

d. Laterally rotates the thigh at the hip joint

e. Medially rotates the thigh at the hip joint

f. Abducts the thigh at the hip joint

g. Adducts the thigh at the hip joint

h. Anteriorly tilts the pelvis

i. Posteriorly tilts the pelvis

j. Contralaterally rotates the pelvis

k. Depresses same-side pelvis

Muscle

1. Gluteus maximus ___ ___ ___ ___ ___ ___

2. Gluteus medius ___ ___ ___ ___ ___ ___ ___ ___

3. Gluteus minimus ___ ___ ___ ___ ___ ___ ___ ___

4. Piriformis ___ ___ ___ ___

5. Superior gemellus ___ ___

6. Obturator internus ___ ___

7. Inferior gemellus ___ ___

8. Obturator externus ___ ___

9. Quadratus femoris ___ ___

Score: ___/38

THE LONG AND THE SHORT OF IT – EXERCISE 1

For each joint action given, indicate whether the muscle shortens or lengthens.

1. Quadratus femoris: ipsilateral rotation of the pelvis: _____

2. Gluteus minimus (posterior fibers): posterior tilt of the pelvis: _____

3. Superior gemellus: medial rotation of the thigh at the hip joint: _____

4. Piriformis: horizontal extension of the thigh at the hip joint: _____

5. Gluteus medius: abduction of the thigh at the hip joint: _____

Score: ___/5

THE LONG AND THE SHORT OF IT – EXERCISE 2

For each joint action given, fill in the blanks with a muscle that shortens and a muscle that lengthens. Please note that possible answers may be covered in another section.

1. Flexes the thigh at the hip joint:

   Shortens: _____   Lengthens: _____

2. Extends the thigh at the hip joint:

   Shortens: _____   Lengthens: _____

Chapter **10** **Muscles of the Pelvis and Thigh**

3. Medially rotates the thigh at the hip joint:

Shortens: _____ Lengthens: _____

4. Adducts the thigh at the hip joint:

Shortens: _____ Lengthens: _____

5. Laterally rotates the thigh at the hip joint:

Shortens: _____ Lengthens: _____

Score: ___/10

MOVERS & ANTAGONISTS – EXERCISE 1

For each joint action stated, fill in the blank for a mover and antagonist of that joint action. Please choose your mover/antagonist pairs from the word bank below. Each pair can be used only once.

Upper gluteus maximus/Lower gluteus maximus

Anterior gluteus medius/Posterior gluteus medius

Gluteus maximus/Anterior gluteus medius

Piriformis/Anterior gluteus minimus

1. Flexes the thigh at the hip joint:

_____

2. Laterally rotates the thigh at the hip joint:

_____

3. Posteriorly tilts the pelvis at the hip joint:

_____

4. Abducts the thigh at the hip joint:

_____

Score: ___/4

For each joint action illustrated, the body part is being *slowly* moved in the direction indicated by the arrow. Circle whether the functional muscle group of the pair provided is contracting or relaxed. Then circle *how* the muscle group that is working is contracting (concentrically or eccentrically).

1.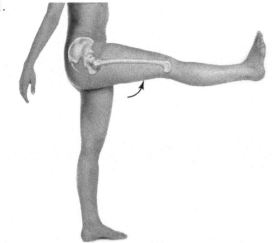

Movement:

Flexion of the thigh at the hip joint

Flexors: contracting/relaxed

Extensors: contracting/relaxed

What type of contraction is occurring?
concentric/eccentric

2.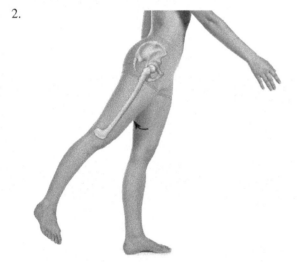

Movement:

Extension of the thigh at the hip joint

Extensors: contracting/relaxed

Flexors: contracting/relaxed

What type of contraction is occurring?
concentric/eccentric

3.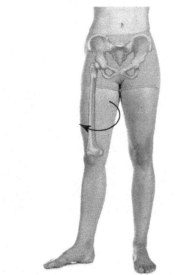

Movement:

Lateral rotation of the thigh at the hip joint

Lateral rotators: contracting/relaxed

Medial rotators: contracting/relaxed

What type of contraction is occurring?
concentric/eccentric

Score: ___/9

Chapter **10** **Muscles of the Pelvis and Thigh**

MUSCLE STABILIZATIONS

Circle the letter of the best answer to the question.

1. Which of the following muscles can stabilize the thigh and pelvis at the hip joint?

    a. Gluteus maximus
    b. Superior gemellus
    c. Obturator internus
    d. All of the above

2. Which of the following muscles can stabilize the sacrum at the sacroiliac joints?

    a. Quadratus femoris
    b. Piriformis
    c. Gluteus medius
    d. Obturator externus

3. Which of the following muscles can stabilize the sacrum at the lumbosacral joints?

    a. Gluteus medius
    b. Quadratus femoris
    c. Gluteus minimus
    d. Piriformis

Score: ___/3

YOU'VE GOT NERVE!

Write in the name of the corresponding innervation from the list provided. Choices can be used more than once.

Inferior gluteal nerve

Superior gluteal nerve

Nerve to piriformis (of the lumbosacral plexus)

Nerve to obturator internus (of the lumbosacral plexus)

Nerve to quadratus femoris (of the lumbosacral plexus)

The obturator nerve

1. Gluteus maximus _____

2. Gluteus medius _____

3. Gluteus minimus _____

4. Piriformis _____

5. Superior gemellus _____

6. Obturator internus _____

7. Inferior gemellus _____

8. Obturator externus _____

9. Quadratus femoris _____

Score: ___/9

ARE YOU FEELING IT? – PALPATION

Fill in the blank with the best answer to the palpation question.

1. What do we ask the client to do to engage and palpate the gluteus maximus?

   _____

2. What is the optimal position in which to palpate the gluteus medius?

   _____

3. Where is the piriformis located?

   _____

4. Where is the quadratus femoris located for palpation?

   _____

5. Where do we add resistance when engaging and palpating the gluteus maximus?

   _____

Score: ___/5

CLINICALLY SPEAKING

Fill in the blank with the best answer for the treatment consideration question.

1. What gluteal muscle usually has a thick layer of fascia over it?

   _____

2. What muscle can be thought of as the "deltoid of the hip joint"?

   _____

3. Standing with all or most of your weight on one foot causes what muscle(s) to work harder?

   _____

4. If the thigh is first flexed to approximately 60 degrees or more, what is the piriformis' transverse plane action at the hip joint?

   _____

5. Approximately 10 to 20 percent of the time, how does the sciatic nerve present?

   _____

6. What name is given to compression of the sciatic nerve caused by the piriformis?

   _____

Score: ___/6

Chapter **10** **Muscles of the Pelvis and Thigh**

Fill in the blank with the best answer to the question.

1. What muscle is known as the speed skater's muscle?

_____

2. What are the names of the three muscles of the gluteal group?

_____

3. What are the names of the muscles of the deep lateral rotator group?

_____

4. What are the two sagittal plane actions of the anterior fibers of the gluteus medius?

_____

5. What is the deepest muscle of the gluteal group?

_____

6. In which region is the gluteus medius superficial?

_____

7. What do all rotators of the thigh at the hip joint do if the thigh is fixed and the pelvis moves instead?

_____

8. What deep lateral rotator attaches to the sacrum?

_____

9. What is the most inferior of the deep lateral rotators?

_____

10. What muscle is superficial to the piriformis?

_____

Score: ___/10

CROSSWORD PUZZLE

Use the clues to complete the crossword puzzle.

ACROSS

4 Reverse actions at the hip joint move the _____
7 Gluteal "deltoid of hip"
9 Gluteus muscle that abducts and adducts
10 _____ internus/externus
12 Sciatic nerve usually passes between piriformis and this gemellus

DOWN

1 Superior and inferior muscle twins
2 Obturator externus' location relative to the quadratus femoris
3 Least
5 Can cause sciatica
6 Square-shaped deep lateral rotator of the femur
8 Distal attachment of gluteus maximus (acronym)
11 Anteriorly, the gluteus medius is deep to this muscle (acronym)

Score: ___/12

Fill in the blank with the best answer for the clinical case study questions.

1. If a client comes in with the iliac crest low on the right and you suspect that the right lower extremity is short, what muscle would you first look to assess?

   _____

2. You assess the client's tight piriformis. How do you stretch it?

   _____

3. When the client walks, you see that her patella turns in as the foot hits the ground. You suspect that this occurs due to the arch on that side collapsing upon weight bearing. Strengthening what musculature do you think might help this client?

   _____

4. A new client presents to you with a spasm in their piriformis. What joint should be assessed?

   _____

Score: ___/4

Section 2 tests your knowledge of muscles covered in pages 356–370 of the *Know the Body* textbook.

KNOW YOUR MUSCLES

Fill in the blank with the name of the muscle being palpated.

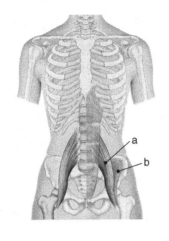
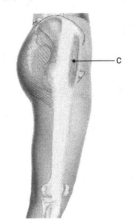
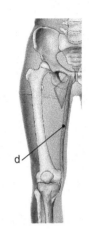

a _____

b _____

c _____

d _____

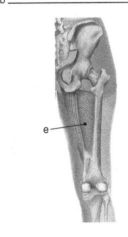
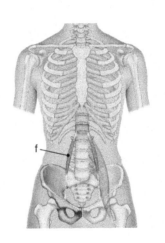
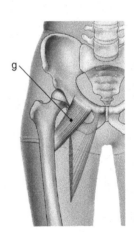

e _____

f _____

g _____

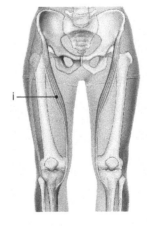

h _____

i _____

Score: ___/9

213

Match the muscle name from the right column to its meaning in the left column. Write your answer in the space provided. Each choice can be used only once.

Meaning

_____ 1. Comb-like appearance

_____ 2. Small muscle of the low back area

_____ 3. Short adductor muscle

_____ 4. Large muscle of the low back area

_____ 5. Muscle attaching to the ilium

_____ 6. Muscle that creates the cross-legged position of a tailor

_____ 7. Large adductor muscle

_____ 8. Long adductor muscle

_____ 9. Slender and graceful shape

_____ 10. Tenses the fascia lata

Muscle name

a. Sartorius

b. Adductor longus

c. Adductor brevis

d. Gracilis

e. Iliacus

f. Adductor magnus

g. Pectineus

h. Psoas major

i. Tensor fasciae latae

j. Psoas minor

Score: ___/10

MATCHING ATTACHMENTS

Match each muscle from the word bank with its attachments. Write the answer in the column labeled *Muscle*. Each choice can be used only once.

Adductor longus   Psoas major

Adductor magnus   Psoas minor

Adductor brevis   Pectineus

Sartorius   Gracilis

Tensor fasciae latae   Iliacus

Attachments	Muscle
1. Anterior superior iliac spine *to the* Iliotibial band	
2. Anterior superior iliac spine *to the* Pes anserine tendon at the proximal anteromedial tibia	
3. Internal ilium *to the* Lesser trochanter of the femur	
4. Anterolateral lumbar spine *to the* Lesser trochanter of the femur	
5. Anterolateral bodies of T12 and L1 *to the* Pubis	

6. Pubis *to the* Proximal posterior shaft of the femur	
7. Pubis *to the* Pes anserine tendon at the proximal anteromedial tibia	
8. Pubis *to the* Linea aspera of the femur	
9. Pubis *to the* Linea aspera of the femur	
10. Pubis and ischium *to the* Linea aspera of the femur	

Score: ___/10

THE BIG PICTURE – FUNCTIONAL GROUPS

Fill in the blanks with 1) the direction of movement, 2) the body part that is moving, and 3) the joint at which movement is occurring.

1. If a muscle crosses the hip joint anteriorly with a vertical direction to its fibers, what two actions can it perform?

   _____ of the _____ at the _____ joint(s).

   _____ of the _____ at the _____ joint(s).

2. If a muscle crosses the hip joint posteriorly with a vertical direction to its fibers, what two actions can it perform?

   _____ of the _____ at the _____ joint(s).

   _____ of the _____ at the _____ joint(s).

3. If a muscle crosses the hip joint laterally with a vertical direction to its fibers, what two actions can it perform?

   _____ of the _____ at the _____ joint(s).

   _____ of the _____ at the _____ joint(s).

4. If a muscle crosses the hip joint medially with a vertical direction to its fibers, what two actions can it perform?

   _____ of the _____ at the _____ joint(s).

   _____ of the _____ at the _____ joint(s).

5. If a muscle crosses the spinal joints of the trunk anteriorly with a vertical direction to its fibers, what action can it perform?

   _____ of the _____ at the _____ joint(s).

6. What is the reverse action of flexion of the thigh at the hip joint?

   _____ of the _____ at the _____ joint(s).

Score: ___/6

215

MATCHING ACTIONS

Place the corresponding joint action letter(s) in the blank(s) next to the muscle. Choices can be used more than once.

a. Flexes the thigh at the hip joint

b. Flexes the leg at the knee joint

c. Flexes the trunk at the lumbar spinal joints

d. Abducts the thigh at the hip joint

e. Adducts the thigh at the hip joint

f. Medially rotates the thigh at the hip joint

g. Laterally rotates the thigh at the hip joint

h. Anteriorly tilts the pelvis

i. Posteriorly tilts the pelvis

j. Depresses the same-side pelvis

k. Extends the thigh at the hip joint

1. Tensor fasciae latae ____ ____ ____ ____ ____

2. Sartorius ____ ____ ____ ____ ____

3. Iliacus ____ ____ ____

4. Psoas major ____ ____ ____ ____

5. Psoas minor ____ ____

6. Pectineus ____ ____ ____

7. Gracilis ____ ____ ____ ____

8. Adductor longus ____ ____ ____

9. Adductor brevis ____ ____ ____

10. Adductor magnus ____ ____ ____

Score: ___/35

THE LONG AND THE SHORT OF IT – EXERCISE 1

For each joint action given, indicate whether the muscle shortens or lengthens.

1. Psoas minor: extension of the trunk at the lumbar spinal joints: _____

2. Adductor longus: anterior tilt of the pelvis: _____

3. Tensor fasciae latae: medial rotation of the thigh at the hip joint: _____

4. Sartorius: flexion of the leg at the knee joint: _____

5. Gracilis: extension of the leg at the knee joint: _____

Score: ___/5

THE LONG AND THE SHORT OF IT – EXERCISE 2

For each joint action given, fill in the blanks with a muscle that shortens and a muscle that lengthens. Please note that possible answers may be covered in another section.

1. Extension of the thigh at the hip joint

   Shortens: _____   Lengthens: _____

2. Anterior tilt of the pelvis

   Shortens: _____   Lengthens: _____

3. Medial rotation of the thigh at the hip joint

Shortens: _____   Lengthens: _____

4. Flexion of the thigh at the hip joint

Shortens: _____   Lengthens: _____

5. Abduction of the thigh at the hip joint

Shortens: _____   Lengthens: _____

Score: ___/10

MOVERS & ANTAGONISTS – EXERCISE 1

For each joint action stated, fill in the blank for a mover and antagonist of that joint action. Please choose your mover/antagonist pairs from the word bank below. Each pair can be used only once.

Adductor magnus/Posterior gluteus medius

Sartorius/Tensor fasciae latae

Gluteus maximus/Iliopsoas

Sartorius/Gluteus maximus

1. Extends the thigh at the hip joint:

_____

2. Laterally rotates thigh at the hip joint:

_____

3. Adducts the thigh at the hip joint:

_____

4. Anteriorly tilts the pelvis at the hip joint:

_____

Score: ___/4

For each joint action illustrated, the body part is being *slowly* moved in the direction indicated by the arrow. Circle whether the functional muscle group of the pair provided is contracting or relaxed. Then circle *how* the muscle group that is working is contracting (concentrically or eccentrically).

1.

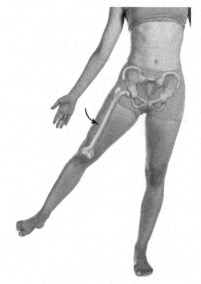

Movement:

Adduction of the thigh at the hip joint

Adductors: contracting/relaxed

Abductors: contracting/relaxed

What type of contraction is occurring?
concentric/eccentric

2.

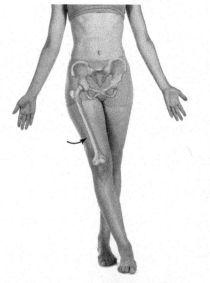

Movement:

Adduction of the thigh at the hip joint

Adductors: contracting/relaxed

Abductors: contracting/relaxed

What type of contraction is occurring?
concentric/eccentric

3.

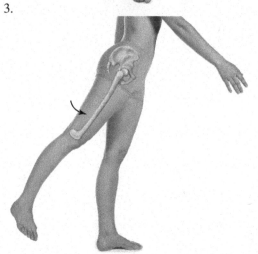

Movement:

Flexion of the thigh at the hip joint

Flexors: contracting/relaxed

Extensors: contracting/relaxed

What type of contraction is occurring?
concentric/eccentric

Score: ___/9

218

Chapter **10** **Muscles of the Pelvis and Thigh**

MUSCLE STABILIZATIONS

Circle the letter of the best answer to the question.

1. Which of the following muscles can stabilize the knee via the iliotibial band?
   a. Tensor fasciae latae
   b. Gracilis
   c. Sartorius
   d. Psoas major

2. Which of the following muscles can stabilize the knee via the Pes anserine tendon?
   a. Gracilis
   b. Adductor magnus
   c. Tensor fasciae latae
   d. Iliacus

3. Which of the following muscles can stabilize the lumbar spinal joints?
   a. Iliacus
   b. Pectineus
   c. Psoas minor
   d. Adductor brevis

4. Which of the following muscles does NOT act to stabilize the knee joint?
   a. Tensor fasciae latae
   b. Adductor longus
   c. Sartorius
   d. Gracilis

Score: ___/4

YOU'VE GOT NERVE!

Write the name of the corresponding innervation(s) from the list provided. Choices can be used more than once.

Superior gluteal nerve

Femoral nerve

Lumbar plexus

L1 spinal nerve

Obturator nerve

Sciatic nerve

1. Tensor fasciae latae _____

2. Sartorius _____

3. Iliacus _____

4. Psoas major _____

5. Psoas minor _____

6. Pectineus _____

7. Gracilis _____

8. Adductor longus _____

9. Adductor brevis _____

10. Adductor magnus _____ & _____

Score: ___/11

ARE YOU FEELING IT? – PALPATION

Fill in the blank with the best answer to the palpation question.

1. What actions do we ask the client to perform to engage and palpate the tensor fasciae latae?

_____

2. What actions do we ask the client to perform to engage and palpate the sartorius?

_____

3. When palpating the tensor fasciae latae or sartorius, where is resistance applied?

_____

4. To palpate the belly of the psoas major in the abdomen, where should the palpating finger pads be placed?

_____

5. Which adductor group tendon is most easily palpable?

_____

6. The adductor magnus is superficial in the medial thigh between which two muscles?

_____

Score: ___/6

CLINICALLY SPEAKING

Fill in the blank with the best answer for the treatment consideration question.

1. What condition can be caused by a tight tensor fasciae latae?

_____

2. Which three muscles attach into the pes anserine tendon?

_____

3. What structures are located in the femoral triangle of the thigh?

_____

4. Caution should be exercised when palpating the psoas major in the abdomen due to the presence of what structure?

_____

5. What two muscles border the femoral triangle?

_____

6. What muscle is sometimes known as the *fourth hamstring*?

_____

Score: ___/6

MUSCLE MASH-UP

Fill in the blank with the best answer to the question.

1. Which two muscles comprise the iliopsoas?

_____

2. What are the names of the five muscles of the adductor group?

_____

3. What is the only member of the adductor group that crosses the knee joint?

_____

4. Which muscle of the adductor group is most posterior?

_____

5. What two muscles attach into the iliotibial band?

_____

6. What is the common origin (proximal attachment) for the adductor group?

_____

7. What muscle crosses spinal joints and the hip joint?

_____

8. Which adductor has a very prominent proximal tendon?

_____

9. What muscle is immediately medial to the iliopsoas in the proximal thigh?

_____

10. What are the two sagittal plane actions of the adductor magnus?

_____

11. What are the two heads of the adductor magnus?

_____

12. What nerves pierce through the belly of the psoas major?

_____

Score: ___/12

MINI CASE STUDIES

Fill in the blank with the best answer for the clinical case study questions.

1. A new client presents with tingling in the proximal lateral thigh. What condition do you suspect? And what muscle would you assess?

_____

2. You palpate and assess a new client's psoas major as tight. As a result of this, what postural condition might you expect to find?

_____

3. A client has limited range of motion of abduction of the thigh at the hip joint. What muscle group should you assess for tightness?

_____

4. What condition do you suspect in a teenage client who has recently had a growth spurt accompanied by tightness and pain in the abdomen?

_____

Score: ___/4

Use the clues to complete the crossword puzzle.

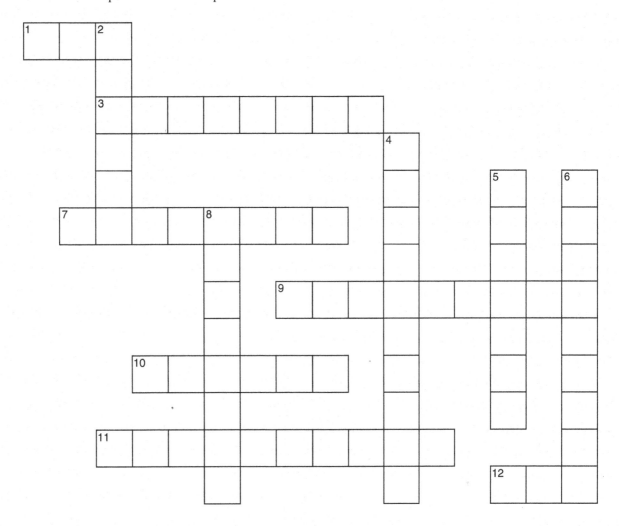

ACROSS

1 Immediately distal and lateral to the ASIS (acronym)
3 Hyperlordosis
7 Slender, graceful
9 Common distal tendon attachment at the proximal anteromedial knee (two words)
10 It is best to keep curl-ups under _____ degrees
11 Filet mignon (two words)
12 Foot

DOWN

2 Trochanter attachment of iliopsoas
4 Muscle that is often absent (two words)
5 Nerve that innervates most of the anterior thigh musculature
6 Crosses the hip joint anteriorly and the knee joint posteriorly
8 This ligament runs superficial to the iliopsoas

Score: ___/12

Section 3 tests your knowledge of muscle covered in pages 372–380 of the *Know the Body* textbook.

KNOW YOUR MUSCLES

Fill in the blank with the name of the muscles shown.

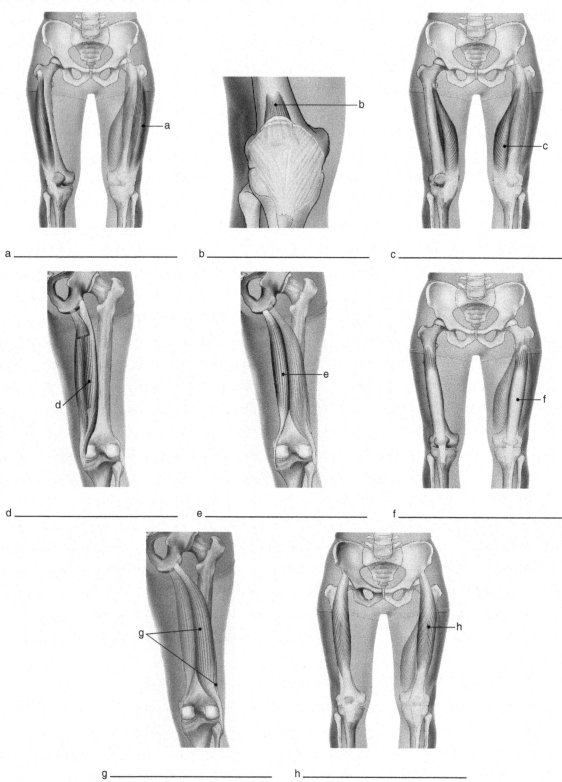

a _____   b _____   c _____

d _____   e _____   f _____

g _____   h _____

Score: ___/8

WHAT'S IN A NAME?

Match the muscle name from the right column to its meaning in the left column. Write your answer in the space provided. Each choice can be used only once.

Meaning

_____ 1. Muscle with a flattened, membranous attachment

_____ 2. Muscle with a long, slender tendon

_____ 3. Two-headed muscle of the femur

_____ 4. Muscle running straight up and down the femur

_____ 5. Large, laterally located muscle

_____ 6. Large muscle located between two other muscles

_____ 7. Large, medially located muscle

_____ 8. Muscle involved with the knee joint

Muscle name

a. Vastus medialis

b. Semimembranosus

c. Semitendinosus

d. Vastus lateralis

e. Articularis genus

f. Rectus femoris

g. Biceps femoris

h. Vastus intermedius

Score: ___/8

MATCHING ATTACHMENTS

Match each muscle from the word bank with its attachments. Write the answer in the column labeled *Muscle*. Each choice will be used only once.

Vastus intermedius	Rectus femoris
Vastus medialis	Biceps femoris
Vastus lateralis	Articularis genus
Semimembranosus	Semitendinosus

Attachments	Muscle
1. Anterior inferior iliac spine *to the* Tibial tuberosity via the patella and the patellar ligament	
2. Linea aspera of the femur *to the* Tibial tuberosity via the patella and the patellar ligament	
3. Linea aspera of the femur *to the* Tibial tuberosity via the patella and the patellar ligament	
4. Anterior shaft and linea aspera of the femur *to the* Tibial tuberosity via the patella and the patellar ligament	
5. Anterior distal femoral shaft *to the* Knee joint capsule	

6. Long Head: Ischial tuberosity
   Short Head: Linea aspera
   to the
   Head of the fibula	

7. Ischial tuberosity
   to the
   Pes anserine tendon (at the proximal anteromedial tibia)	

8. Ischial tuberosity
   to the
   Posterior surface of the medial condyle of the tibia	

Score: ___/8

THE BIG PICTURE – FUNCTIONAL GROUPS

Fill in the blanks with 1) the direction of movement, 2) the body part that is moving, and 3) the joint at which movement is occurring.

1. If a muscle crosses the hip joint anteriorly with a vertical direction to its fibers, what two actions can it perform?

   _____ of the _____ at the _____ joint(s).

   _____ of the _____ at the _____ joint(s).

2. If a muscle crosses the hip joint posteriorly with a vertical direction to its fibers, what two actions can it perform?

   _____ of the _____ at the _____ joint(s).

   _____ of the _____ at the _____ joint(s).

3. If a muscle crosses the knee joint anteriorly with a vertical direction to its fibers, what action can it perform?

   _____ of the _____ at the _____ joint(s).

4. If a muscle crosses the knee joint posteriorly with a vertical direction to its fibers, what action can it perform?

   _____ of the _____ at the _____ joint(s).

5. What is the reverse action of flexion of the thigh at the hip joint?

   _____ of the _____ at the _____ joint(s).

6. What is the reverse action of extension of the leg at the knee joint?

   _____ of the _____ at the _____ joint(s).

Score: ___/6

MATCHING ACTIONS

Place the corresponding joint action letter(s) in the blank(s) next to the muscle. The number of blanks next to each muscle name indicates the number of letters that should be placed next to that muscle.

Joint Action

a. Extends the leg at the knee joint

b. Extends the thigh at the knee joint

c. Extends the thigh at the hip joint

d. Flexes the thigh at the hip joint

e. Flexes the leg at the knee joint

f. Anteriorly tilts the pelvis

g. Posteriorly tilts the pelvis

h. Proximally tenses and pulls the knee joint capsule

Muscle

1. Rectus femoris ____ ____ ____ ____

2. Vastus lateralis ____ ____

3. Vastus medialis ____ ____

4. Vastus intermedius ____ ____

5. Articularis genus ____

6. Biceps femoris ____ ____ ____

7. Semitendinosus ____ ____ ____

8. Semimembranosus ____ ____ ____

Score: ___/20

THE LONG AND THE SHORT OF IT – EXERCISE 1

For each joint action given, indicate whether the muscle shortens or lengthens.

1. Vastus lateralis: extension of the leg at the knee joint: _____

2. Semitendinosus: extension of the thigh at the hip joint: _____

3. Articularis genus: the knee joint capsule moves distally: _____

4. Rectus femoris: anterior tilt of the pelvis: _____

5. Vastus intermedius: flexion of the leg at the knee joint: _____

Score: ___/5

THE LONG AND THE SHORT OF IT – EXERCISE 2

For each joint action given, fill in the blanks with a muscle that shortens and a muscle that lengthens. Please note that possible answers may be covered in another section.

1. Extension of the leg at the knee joint

   Shortens: _____ Lengthens: _____

2. Posterior tilt of the pelvis

   Shortens: _____ Lengthens: _____

3. Flexion of the thigh at the hip joint

   Shortens: _____ Lengthens: _____

4. Flexion of the leg at the knee joint

   Shortens: _____ Lengthens: _____

5. Anterior tilt of the pelvis at the hip joint

   Shortens: _____ Lengthens: _____

MOVERS & ANTAGONISTS – EXERCISE 1

For each joint action stated, fill in the blank for a mover and antagonist of that joint action. Please choose your mover/antagonist pairs from the word bank below. Each pair can be used once and only once.

Rectus femoris/Gluteus maximus

Hamstring group/Quadriceps femoris group

Biceps femoris/Iliopsoas

Vastus lateralis/Semitendinosus

1. Flexes the leg at the knee joint:

   _____

2. Extends the thigh at the knee joint:

   _____

3. Anteriorly tilts the pelvis at the hip joint:

   _____

4. Extends the thigh at the hip joint:

   _____

For each joint action illustrated, the body part is being *slowly* moved in the direction indicated by the arrow. Circle whether the functional muscle group of the pair provided is contracting or relaxed. Then circle *how* the muscle group that is working is contracting (concentrically or eccentrically).

1.

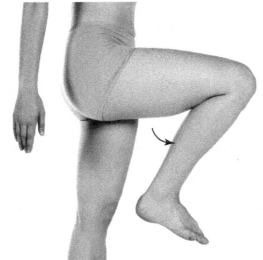

Movement:

Extension of the leg at the knee joint

   Extensors: contracting/relaxed

   Flexors: contracting/relaxed

   What type of contraction is occurring?
   concentric/eccentric

2.

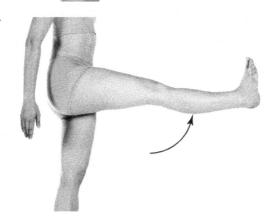

Movement:

Extension of the leg at the knee joint

   Extensors: contracting/relaxed

   Flexors: contracting/relaxed

   What type of contraction is occurring?
   concentric/eccentric

3.

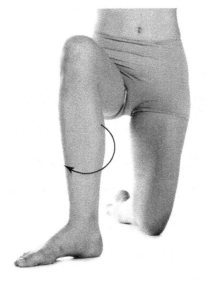

Movement:

Lateral rotation of the leg at the knee joint

   Lateral rotators: contracting/relaxed

   Medial rotators: contracting/relaxed

   What type of contraction is occurring?
   concentric/eccentric

Score: ___/9

229

MUSCLE STABILIZATIONS

Circle the letter of the best answer to the question.

1. Which of the following muscles stabilizes both the pelvis AND the knee joint?
   a. Vastus lateralis
   b. Vastus medialis
   c. Rectus femoris
   d. Articularis genus

2. Which of the following muscles stabilizes only the knee joint?
   a. Biceps femoris
   b. Semimembranosus
   c. Rectus femoris
   d. Vastus intermedius

3. Which of the following muscles stabilizes the position of the knee joint capsule?
   a. Articularis genus
   b. Semitendinosus
   c. Vastus lateralis
   d. Biceps femoris

Score: ___/3

YOU'VE GOT NERVE!

Write the name of the corresponding innervation from the list provided.

Femoral nerve

Sciatic nerve

1. Rectus femoris _____

2. Vastus lateralis _____

3. Vastus medialis _____

4. Vastus intermedius _____

5. Articularis genus _____

6. Biceps femoris _____

7. Semitendinosus _____

8. Semimembranosus _____

Score: ___/8

ARE YOU FEELING IT? – PALPATION

Fill in the blank with the best answer to the palpation question.

1. What joint action will engage all four quadriceps femoris muscles for palpation?

_____

2. What is the bony landmark that should be found to begin palpating the hamstrings proximally?

_____

3. When palpating the quadriceps femoris group, where is resistance applied?

_____

4. What muscle can be palpated deep to the iliotibial band?

_____

5. What joint action should the client perform to engage and palpate the hamstrings?

_____

6. At what bony landmark can the distal tendon of the biceps femoris be palpated?

_____

Score: ___/6

CLINICALLY SPEAKING

Fill in the blank with the best answer for the treatment consideration question.

1. Which three muscles attach into the pes anserine tendon?

_____

2. What muscle is named for its long distal tendon?

_____

3. What muscle is named for its long flattened proximal tendon?

_____

4. What is the largest part of the vastus medialis?

_____

5. Pain in the lateral thigh is often attributed to the iliotibial band, when often it is actually caused by what muscle?

_____

Score: ___/5

Fill in the blank with the best answer to the question.

1. What are the names of the four quadriceps femoris muscles?

   _____

2. What are the three hamstring muscles?

   _____

3. What are the medial hamstrings?

   _____

4. What are the two heads of the biceps femoris?

   _____

5. What muscle contracts to pull the knee joint capsule proximally?

   _____

6. Common proximal attachment for the hamstrings.

   _____

7. What is the only quadriceps femoris muscle to cross the hip joint?

   _____

8. What is the only hamstring muscle/head that does NOT cross the hip joint?

   _____

9. What is the largest quadriceps femoris muscle?

   _____

10. What quadriceps femoris muscle is most difficult to palpate?

    _____

11. What is the common origin (proximal attachment) for the three vastus muscles of the quadriceps group?

    _____

12. Which medial hamstring is deeper?

    _____

Score: ___/12

Use the clues to complete the crossword puzzle.

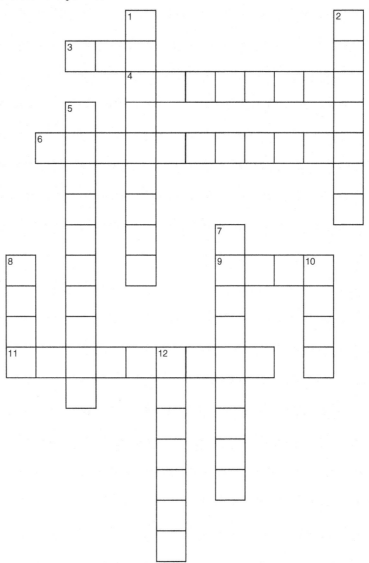

ACROSS

3 Lower fibers of the vastus medialis (acronym)
4 Rectus
6 Location of biceps femoris long head compared to short head
9 Origin (proximal attachment) of rectus femoris (acronym)
11 Quadriceps femoris joint action of the knee

DOWN

1 Direction of hamstrings' tilt action on pelvis
2 Bone located within quadriceps femoris distal tendon
5 Common tibial attachment for quadriceps femoris
7 Directly medial to rectus femoris in the proximal thigh
8 Genu
10 Beginning of name for both medial hamstrings
12 Innervation to the hamstrings

Score: ___/12

233

MINI CASE STUDIES

Fill in the blank with the best answer for the clinical case study questions.

1. A new client's former therapist told him he has iliotibial band tightness and pain. What muscles should you assess?

   _____

2. A client is experiencing general knee joint weakness and discomfort. What muscle group is probably most important to strengthen?

   _____

3. A new client is very restricted in flexion of the thigh at the hip joint range of motion if the knee joint is extended. What muscles should be worked?

   _____

4. If a client is experiencing medial meniscus problems, which hamstring is probably most important to work?

   _____

Score: ___/4

MNEMONICS

Create your own mnemonic for the muscle group.

Pes anserine muscles:

Sartorius, Gracilis, SemiTendinosus

Sensitive Guys Smile Tenderly!

Now make one of your own:

S _____ G _____ S _____ T _____.

Adductor group:

Pectineus, Gracilis, (Adductor) Longus, Brevis, Magnus

Pretty Girls Love Big Muscles!

Now make one of your own:

P _____ G _____ L _____ B _____ M _____.

Quadriceps femoris muscles:

Rectus Femoris, Vastus Medialis, Vastus Intermedius, Vastus Lateralis

Robert's Family, Very Musical, Very Interesting, Very Loud!

Now make one of your own:

R _____ F _____ V _____ M _____ V _____

I _____ V _____ L _____.

Hamstring muscles:

Biceps Femoris, SemiTendinosus, SemiMembranosus

Big Fables Sometimes Tell Silly Morals!

Now make one of your own:

B _____ F _____ S _____ T _____ S _____

M _____.

11 Muscles of the Leg and Foot

COLORING & LABELING

Use crayons or felt-tipped markers to color the muscles. Use the word banks to fill in the numbers that correspond to the names of the muscles in the blanks provided.

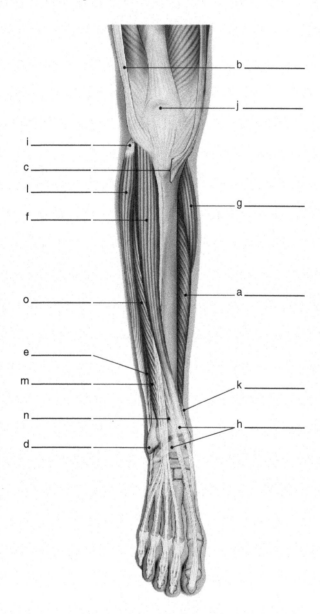

1. Extensor digitorum longus	6. Flexor digitorum longus	11. Patella
2. Extensor hallucis longus	7. Gastrocnemius medial head	12. Pes anserine tendon
3. Fibularis brevis	8. Head of fibula	13. Soleus
4. Fibularis longus	9. Iliotibial band	14. Superior and inferior extensor retinacula
5. Fibularis tertius	10. Lateral malleolus of fibula	15. Tibialis anterior

Score: ___/15

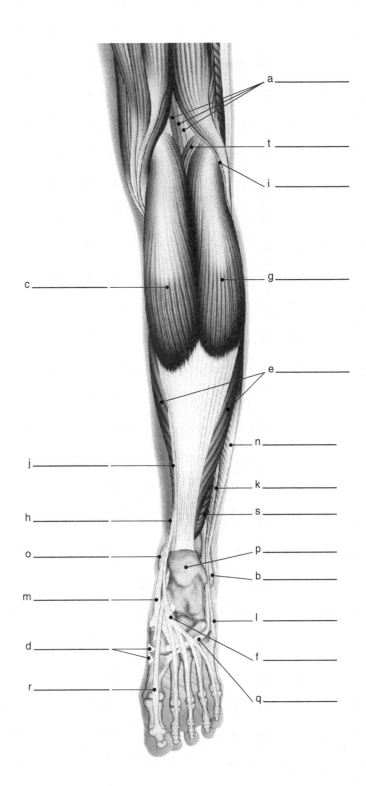

a _____

t _____

i _____

c _____   g _____

e _____

j _____   n _____

k _____

h _____   s _____

o _____   p _____

b _____

m _____   l _____

d _____   f _____

r _____   q _____

1. Calcaneus
2. Common fibular nerve
3. Femoral artery and vein, tibial nerve
4. Fibularis brevis
5. Fibularis brevis tendon

6. Fibularis longus
7. Fibularis longus tendon
8. Flexor digitorum longus
9. Flexor digitorum longus tendon
10. Flexor hallucis longus

11. Flexor hallucis longus
12. Gastrocnemius lateral head
13. Gastrocnemius medial head
14. Lateral malleolus of fibula
15. Medial malleolus of tibia

16. Plantaris
17. Plantaris tendon
18. Soleus
19. Tibialis anterior
20. Tibialis posterior

Score: ___/20

Chapter **11** **Muscles of the Leg and Foot**

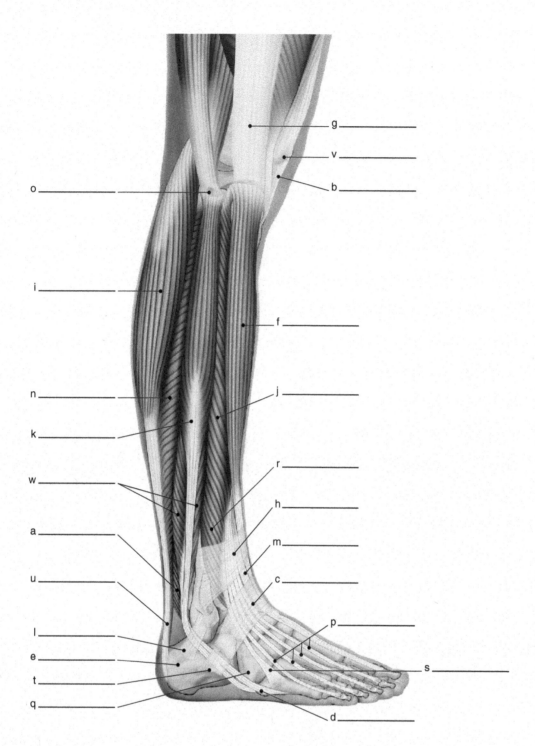

g _____

v _____

b _____

o _____

i _____

f _____

n _____

j _____

k _____

r _____

w _____

h _____

a _____

m _____

u _____

c _____

p _____

l _____

e _____

s _____

t _____

q _____

d _____

1. Calcaneal (Achilles) tendon
2. Calcaneus
3. Cuboid
4. Extensor digitorum longus
5. Extensor digitorum longus tendons
6. Extensor hallucis longus tendon

7. Fibularis brevis
8. Fibularis brevis tendon
9. Fibularis longus
10. Fibularis tertius
11. Fibularis tertius tendon
12. Flexor hallucis longus

13. Gastrocnemius lateral head
14. Head of fibula
15. Iliotibial band
16. Inferior extensor retinaculum
17. Inferior fibular retinaculum
18. Patella

19. Patellar (Infrapatellar) ligament
20. Soleus
21. Superior extensor retinaculum
22. Superior fibular retinaculum
23. Tibialis anterior

Score: ___/23

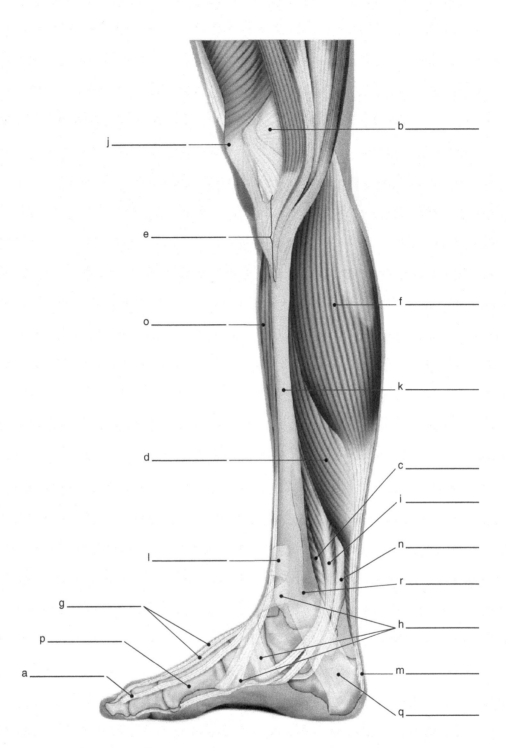

1. 1st metatarsal
2. Calcaneal (Achilles) tendon
3. Extensor digitorum longus tendons
4. Extensor hallucis longus tendon
5. Flexor digitorum longus
6. Flexor hallucis longus

7. Flexor retinaculum
8. Gastrocnemius medial head
9. Inferior extensor retinaculum
10. Medial malleolus of tibia
11. Patella
12. Pes anserine tendon

13. Retinacular fibers
14. Soleus
15. Superior extensor retinaculum
16. Tibia
17. Tibialis anterior
18. Tibialis posterior

Score: ___/18

239

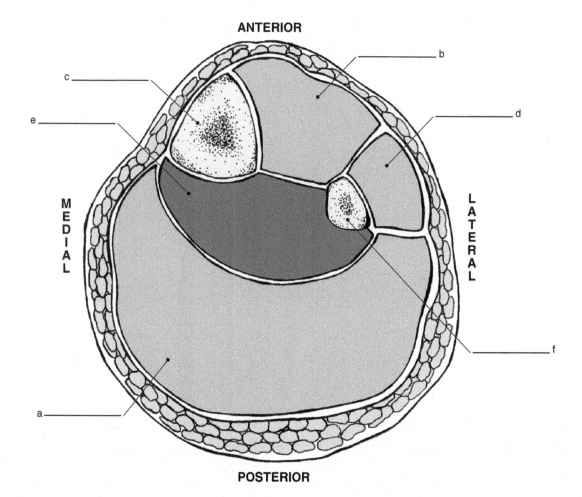

ANTERIOR

MEDIAL

LATERAL

POSTERIOR

c

e

a

b

d

f

1. Anterior compartment

2. Deep posterior compartment

3. Fibula

4. Lateral compartment

5. Superficial posterior compartment

6. Tibia

Anterior compartment:

Tibialis anterior
Extensor digitorum longus
Extensor hallucis longus
Fibularis tertius

Lateral compartment:

Fibularis longus
Fibularis brevis

Superficial posterior compartment:

Gastrocnemius
Soleus
Plantaris

Deep posterior compartment:

Popliteus
Tibialis posterior
Flexor digitorum longus
Flexor hallucis longus

Score: ___/6

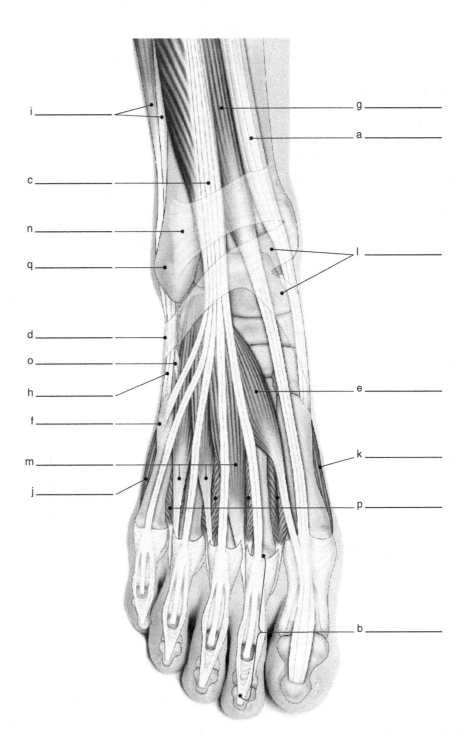

1. Abductor digiti minimi pedis
2. Abductor hallucis
3. Base of 5th metatarsal
4. Dorsal digital expansion of 2nd toe
5. Dorsal interossei pedis
6. Extensor digitorum brevis
7. Extensor digitorum longus and fibularis tertius
8. Extensor hallucis brevis
9. Extensor hallucis longus
10. Fibularis brevis tendon
11. Fibularis longus and brevis
12. Fibularis longus tendon
13. Inferior extensor retinaculum
14. Inferior fibular retinaculum
15. Lateral malleolus of fibula
16. Superior extensor retinaculum
17. Tibialis anterior

Score: ___/17

241

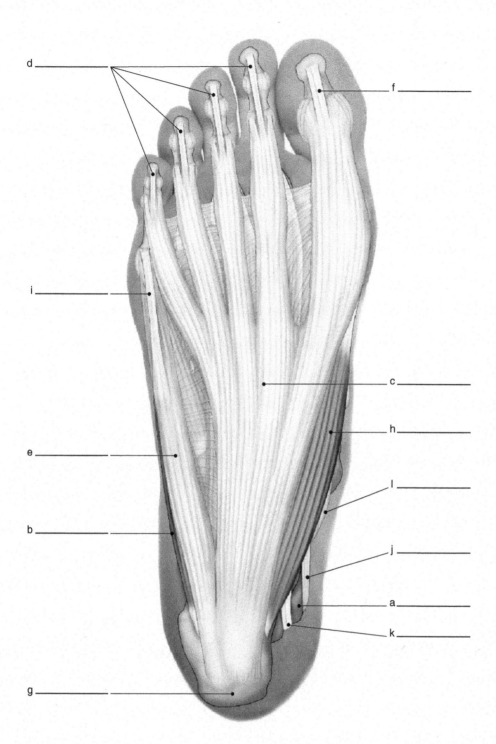

1. Abductor digiti minimi pedis
2. Abductor digiti minimi pedis tendon
3. Abductor hallucis
4. Calcaneus
5. Flexor digitorum longus tendon
6. Flexor digitorum longus tendon
7. Flexor hallucis longus tendon
8. Flexor hallucis longus tendon
9. Lateral plantar fascia
10. Plantar aponeurosis (fascia)
11. Talus
12. Tibialis posterior tendon

Score: ___/12

Section 1 tests your knowledge of the muscles covered in pages 394–402 of the *Know the Body* textbook.

KNOW YOUR MUSCLES

Fill in the blank with the name of the muscles shown.

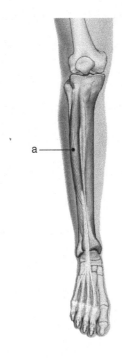

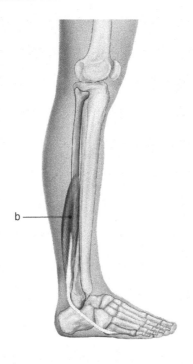

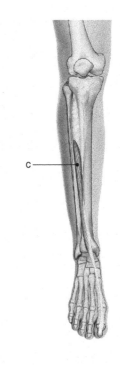

a _____

b _____

c _____

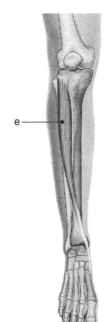

e

f

d _____

e _____

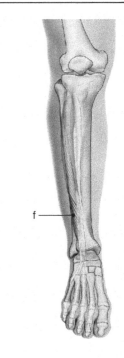

f _____

Score: ___/6

WHAT'S IN A NAME?

Match the muscle name from the right column to its meaning in the left column. Write your answer in the space provided. Each choice can be used only once.

Meaning

_____ 1. Longer muscle that extends the digits

_____ 2. Shorter muscle attaching to the fibula

_____ 3. Third muscle attaching to the fibula

_____ 4. Longer muscle that extends the big toe

_____ 5. Muscle of the anterior tibia

_____ 6. Longer muscle attaching to the fibula

Muscle name

a. Fibularis tertius

b. Fibularis brevis

c. Tibialis anterior

d. Fibularis longus

e. Extensor hallucis longus

f. Extensor digitorum longus

Score: ___/6

MATCHING ATTACHMENTS

Match each muscle from the word bank with its attachments. Write the answer in the column labeled *Muscle*. Each choice can be used only once.

Extensor digitorum longus   Extensor hallucis longus

Tibialis anterior   Fibularis tertius

Fibularis longus   Fibularis brevis

Attachments	Muscle
1. Anterior tibia *to the* Medial foot	
2. Middle anterior fibula *to the* Dorsal surface of the big toe (toe 1)	
3. Proximal anterior fibula *to the* Dorsal surface of toes 2 through 5	
4. Proximal lateral fibula *to the* Medial foot	
5. Distal lateral fibula *to the* Fifth metatarsal	
6. Distal anterior fibula *to the* 5th metatarsal	

Score: ___/6

THE BIG PICTURE – FUNCTIONAL GROUPS

Fill in the blanks with 1) the direction of movement, 2) the body part that is moving, and 3) the joint at which movement is occurring.

1. If a muscle crosses the ankle joint anteriorly with a vertical direction to its fibers, what action can it perform?

   _____ of the _____ at the _____ joint(s).

2. If a muscle crosses the ankle joint posteriorly with a vertical direction to its fibers, what action can it perform?

   _____ of the _____ at the _____ joint(s).

3. If a muscle crosses the subtalar joint medially with a vertical direction to its fibers, what action can it perform?

   _____ of the _____ at the _____ joint(s).

4. If a muscle crosses the subtalar joint laterally with a vertical direction to its fibers, what action can it perform?

   _____ of the _____ at the _____ joint(s).

5. What are reverse actions at the ankle joint?

   _____

   Score: ___/15

MATCHING ACTIONS

Place the corresponding joint action letter(s) in the blank(s) next to the muscle. Choices can be used more than once. The number of blanks next to each muscle name indicates the number of letters that should be placed next to that muscle.

Joint Action

a. Dorsiflexes the foot at the ankle joint

b. Plantarflexes the foot at the ankle joint

c. Inverts the foot at the subtalar joint

d. Everts the foot at the subtalar joint

e. Extends the big toe

f. Extends toes 2 through 5 at the metatarsophalangeal and interphalangeal joints

Muscle

1. Tibialis anterior ____ ____

2. Extensor hallucis longus ____ ____ ____

3. Extensor digitorum longus ____ ____

4. Fibularis longus ____ ____

5. Fibularis brevis ____ ____

6. Fibularis tertius ____ ____

   Score: ___/13

THE LONG AND THE SHORT OF IT – EXERCISE 1

For each joint action given, indicate whether the muscle shortens or lengthens.

1. Tibialis anterior: eversion of the foot at the subtalar joint: _____

2. Extensor digitorum longus: inversion of the foot at the subtalar joint: _____

3. Fibularis tertius: dorsiflexion of the foot at the ankle joint: _____

4. Fibularis longus: dorsiflexion of the foot at the ankle joint: _____

5. Fibularis brevis: eversion of the foot at the subtalar joint: _____

   Score: ___/5

245

For each joint action given, fill in the blanks with a muscle that shortens and a muscle that lengthens. Please note that possible answers may be covered in another section.

1. Eversion of the foot at the subtalar joint

    Shortens: _____   Lengthens: _____

2. Inversion of the foot at the subtalar joint

    Shortens: _____   Lengthens: _____

3. Dorsiflexion of the foot at the ankle joint

    Shortens: _____   Lengthens: _____

4. Plantarflexion of the foot at the ankle joint

    Shortens: _____   Lengthens: _____

5. Extension of the big toe at the
   metatarsophalangeal joint

    Shortens: _____   Lengthens: _____

Score: ___/10

MOVERS & ANTAGONISTS – EXERCISE 1

For each joint action stated, fill in the blank for a mover and antagonist of that joint action. Please choose your mover/antagonist pairs from the word bank below. Each pair can be used only once.

Fibularis longus/Tibialis anterior

Extensor hallucis longus/Fibularis tertius

Fibularis brevis/Extensor digitorum longus

Tibialis anterior/Fibularis longus

1. Dorsiflexes the foot at the ankle joint:

   _____

2. Everts the foot at the subtalar joint:

   _____

3. Plantarflexes the foot at the subtalar joint:

   _____

4. Inverts the foot at the subtalar joint:

   _____

Score: ___/4

For each joint action illustrated, the body part is being *slowly* moved in the direction indicated by the arrow. Circle whether the functional muscle group of the pair provided is contracting or relaxed. Then circle *how* the muscle group that is working is contracting (concentrically or eccentrically.)

1.

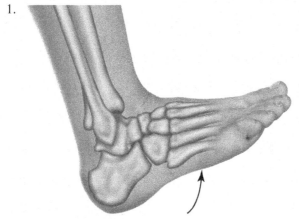

Movement:

Dorsiflexion of the foot at the ankle joint

Dorsiflexors: contracting/relaxed

Plantarflexors: contracting/relaxed

What type of contraction is occurring?
concentric/eccentric

2.

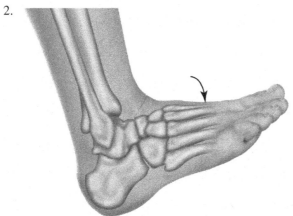

Movement:

Plantarflexion of the foot at the ankle joint

Plantarflexors: contracting/relaxed

Dorsiflexors: contracting/relaxed

What type of contraction is occurring?
concentric/eccentric

3.

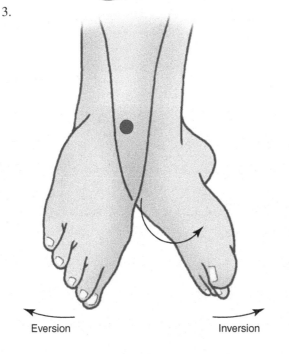

Eversion   Inversion

Movement:

Inversion of the foot at the subtalar joint

Inverters: contracting/relaxed

Everters: contracting/relaxed

What type of contraction is occurring?
concentric/eccentric

Score: ___/9

247

MUSCLE STABILIZATIONS

Circle the letter of the best answer to the question.

1. Which of the following muscles can stabilize the ankle and subtalar joints?
   a. Tibialis anterior
   b. Extensor hallucis longus
   c. Fibularis tertius
   d. All of the above

2. Which of the following muscles can stabilize the metatarsophalangeal joint of the big toe?
   a. Fibularis tertius
   b. Extensor hallucis longus
   c. Tibialis anterior
   d. Extensor digitorum longus

3. Which of the following muscles can stabilize the metatarsophalangeal and interphalangeal joint of toes 2 through 5?
   a. Fibularis longus
   b. Extensor hallucis longus
   c. Fibularis brevis
   d. Extensor digitorum longus

4. Which of the following muscles can stabilize the interphalangeal joint of the big toe?
   a. Fibularis brevis
   b. Extensor digitorum longus
   c. Fibularis tertius
   d. None of the above

Score: ___/4

YOU'VE GOT NERVE!

Write in the name of the corresponding innervation from the list provided.

Deep fibular nerve

Superficial fibular nerve

1. Tibialis anterior _____

2. Extensor hallucis longus _____

3. Extensor digitorum longus _____

4. Fibularis longus _____

5. Fibularis brevis _____

6. Fibularis tertius _____

Score: ___/6

ARE YOU FEELING IT? – PALPATION

Fill in the blank with the best answer to the palpation question.

1. To palpate the tibialis anterior which two actions do you ask the client to perform?

   _____

   _____

2. When engaging and palpating the extensor hallucis longus, resistance should be applied here.

   _____

3. While palpating the extensor digitorum longus, if the client cannot isolate contraction of toes 2 through 5 and therefore also engages and extends the big toe, is it helpful to resist the motion of the client's big toe? Why?

   _____

4. What action do you ask the client to perform in order to engage and palpate the fibularis longus?

   _____

5. How do you find the fibularis tertius?

   _____

   _____

Score: ___/5

CLINICALLY SPEAKING

Fill in the blank with the best answer for the treatment consideration question.

1. What is the most prominent tendon on the dorsal surface of the ankle joint?

   _____

2. What muscle is involved in anterior shin splints?

   _____

3. The fibularis tertius is the most distal and lateral part of what muscle?

   _____

4. What muscle's distal tendon enters the foot on the lateral side, and then travels under the foot to attach to the medial side of the foot?

   _____

Score: ___/5

Fill in the blank with the best answer to the question.

1. What are the names of the three fibularis muscles?

_____

2. What muscle dorsiflexes and inverts the foot?

_____

3. What two muscles evert and plantarflex the foot?

_____

4. Name the four muscles in the anterior compartment of the leg.

_____

5. Name the two muscles in the lateral compartment of the leg.

_____

6. Of the anterior compartment of the leg muscles, which one is deepest?

_____

7. Name a muscle whose distal tendon crosses posterior to the lateral malleolus.

_____

8. What are the names of the two stirrup muscles?

_____

9. All three muscles of this group evert the foot.

_____

10. What muscle's distal tendon becomes the dorsal digital expansion of the foot?

_____

Score: ___/10

Fill in the blank with the best answer for the clinical case study questions.

1. A client has decided to train for a marathon and has recently been running more than usual. She is experiencing pain in the anterior leg that is especially painful upon heel-strike when running. What condition to you suspect and what muscle do you assess?

_____

2. During the history taking with a new client, you discover that the client has had multiple inversion ankle sprains in the past. The strengthening of what muscle group would likely benefit the client.

_____

3. If a client has limited eversion range of motion of the foot, working and loosening what functional group of muscles would likely benefit the client?

_____

4. You note on physical assessment that a client's arch collapses upon weight-bearing. Which two muscles should be strengthened to help support the arch?

_____

_____

Score: ___/4

Use the clues to complete the crossword puzzle.

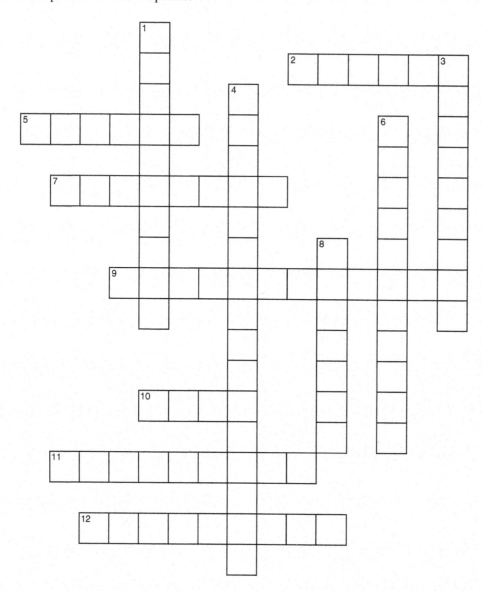

ACROSS

2 Fibularis muscle with a tendon that runs deep in the plantar foot
5 Deeper fibularis muscle
7 Big toe
9 Sagittal plane ankle joint action of extensor digitorum longus
10 During the swing phase of the _____ cycle, we extend our toes so they don't drag on the ground
11 Peroneus
12 Attaches to toes 2 through 5

DOWN

1 Distal attachment of tibialis anterior and fibularis longus (two words)
3 Best position to palpate the fibularis muscles
4 Directly lateral to the tibial shaft in the anterior leg (two words)
6 What nerve innervates the muscles of the anterior compartment? (two words)
8 Third

Score: ___/12

Chapter **11**   **Muscles of the Leg and Foot**

Section 2 tests your knowledge of the muscles covered in pages 404–415 of the *Know the Body* textbook.

KNOW YOUR MUSCLES

Fill in the blank with the name of the muscles shown.

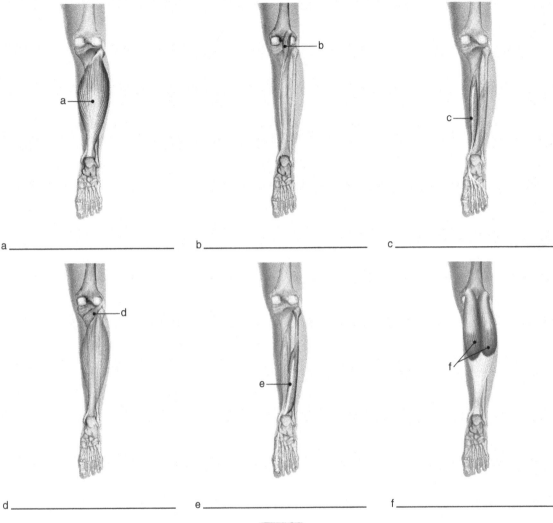

a _____

b _____

c _____

d _____

e _____

f _____

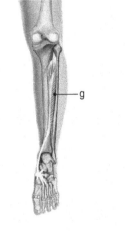

g _____

Score: ___/7

Match the muscle name from the right column to its meaning in the left column. Write your answer in the space provided. Each choice will be used only once.

Meaning

_____ 1. Long muscle that flexes the big toe

_____ 2. Long muscle that flexes the digits

_____ 3. Gives the posterior leg its belly shape

_____ 4. Attaches to the sole of the foot

_____ 5. Located in the posterior knee

_____ 6. Muscle attached to the tibia in the posterior leg

_____ 7. Muscle attached to the bone of the plantar surface of the foot

Muscle name

a. Tibialis posterior

b. Flexor hallucis longus

c. Popliteus

d. Plantaris

e. Flexor digitorum longus

f. Soleus

g. Gastrocnemius

Score: ___/7

MATCHING ATTACHMENTS

Match each muscle from the word bank with its attachments. Write the answer in the column labeled *Muscle*. Each choice will be used only once.

Flexor digitorum longus   Flexor hallucis longus

Tibialis posterior   Gastrocnemius

Plantaris   Popliteus

Soleus

Attachments	Muscle
1. Medial and lateral femoral condyles *to the* Calcaneus via the calcaneal (Achilles) tendon	
2. Posterior tibia and fibula *to the* Calcaneus via the calcaneal (Achilles) tendon	
3. Distal posterolateral femur *to the* Calcaneus	
4. Posterior tibia and fibula *to the* Navicular tuberosity	
5. Middle posterior tibia *to the* Plantar surface of toes 2 through 5	
6. Distal posterior fibula *to the* Plantar surface of the big toe (toe one)	
7. Distal posterolateral femur *to the* Proximal posteromedial tibia	

Score: ___/7

THE BIG PICTURE – FUNCTIONAL GROUPS

Fill in the blanks with 1) the direction of movement, 2) the body part that is moving, and 3) the joint at which movement is occurring.

1. If a muscle crosses the ankle joint posteriorly with a vertical direction to its fibers, what action can it perform?

   _____ of the _____ at the _____ joint(s).

2. If a muscle crosses the subtalar joint medially with a vertical direction to its fibers, what action can it perform?

   _____ of the _____ at the _____ joint(s).

3. If a muscle crosses the knee joint posteriorly with a vertical direction to its fibers, what action can it perform?

   _____ of the _____ at the _____ joint(s).

4. If a muscle crosses toe joints on the plantar side, what action can it perform?

   _____ of the _____.

5. If a muscle crosses toe joints on the dorsal side, what action can it perform?

   _____ of the _____.

6. What is the reverse action of dorsiflexion of the foot at the ankle joint?

   _____ of the _____ at the _____ joint(s).

Score: ___/6

MATCHING ACTIONS

Place the corresponding joint action letter(s) in the blank(s) next to the muscle. Choices can be used more than once. The number of blanks next to each muscle name indicates the number of letters that should be placed next to that muscle.

Joint Action

a. Plantarflexes the foot at the ankle joint

b. Flexes the leg at the knee joint

c. Inverts the foot at the subtalar joint

d. Flexes toes 2 through 5 at the metatarsophalangeal and interphalangeal joint

e. Flexes the big toe at the metatarsophalangeal and interphalangeal joints

f. Medially rotates the leg at the knee joint

g. Laterally rotates the thigh at the knee joint

Muscle

1. Gastrocnemius ____ ____

2. Soleus ____

3. Plantaris ____ ____

4. Tibialis posterior ____ ____

5. Flexor digitorum longus ____ ____ ____

6. Flexor hallucis longus ____ ____ ____

7. Popliteus ____ ____ ____

Score: ___/16

255

THE LONG AND THE SHORT OF IT – EXERCISE 1

For each joint action given, indicate whether the muscle shortens or lengthens.

1. Gastrocnemius: extension of the leg at the knee joint: _____

2. Popliteus: lateral rotation of the thigh at the knee joint: _____

3. Tibialis posterior: plantarflexion of the foot at the ankle joint: _____

4. Soleus: dorsiflexion of the foot at the ankle joint: _____

5. Flexor digitorum longus: eversion of the foot at the subtalar joint: _____

Score: ___/5

THE LONG AND THE SHORT OF IT – EXERCISE 2

For each joint action given, fill in the blanks with a muscle that shortens and a muscle that lengthens. Please note that possible answers may be covered in another section.

1. Medial rotation of the leg at the knee joint

   Shortens: _____

2. Dorsiflexion of the foot at the ankle joint

   Shortens: _____   Lengthens: _____

3. Flexion of toes 2 through 5

   Shortens: _____   Lengthens: _____

4. Flexion of the big toe

   Shortens: _____   Lengthens: _____

5. Inversion of the foot at the subtalar joint

   Shortens: _____   Lengthens: _____

Score: ___/9

For each joint action stated, fill in the blank for a mover and antagonist of that joint action. Please choose your mover/antagonist pairs from the word bank below. Each pair can be used only once.

Tibialis posterior/Fibularis longus

Extensor digitorum longus/Flexor digitorum longus

Gastrocnemius/Tibialis anterior

Extensor hallucis longus/Flexor hallucis longus

1. Plantarflexes the foot at the ankle joint:

2. Extends toes 2 through 5 at the metatarsophalangeal joints:

3. Inverts the foot at the subtalar joint:

4. Extends the big toe at the metatarsophalangeal joint:

Score: ___/4

For each joint action illustrated in which the body part is being *slowly* moved, circle whether the functional muscle group of the pair provided is contracting or relaxed. Then circle *how* the muscle group that is working is contracting (concentrically or eccentrically.)

1.

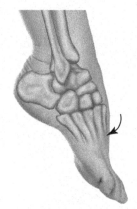

Movement:

Plantarflexion of the foot at the ankle joint

Plantarflexors: contracting/relaxed

Dorsiflexors: contracting/relaxed

What type of contraction is occurring?
concentric/eccentric

2.

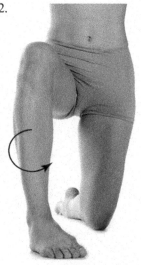

Movement:

Medial rotation of the leg at the knee joint

Medial rotators: contracting/relaxed

Lateral rotators: contracting/relaxed

What type of contraction is occurring?
concentric/eccentric

3.

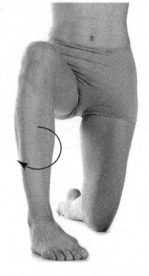

Movement:

Lateral rotation of the leg at the knee joint

Lateral rotators: contracting/relaxed

Medial rotators: contracting/relaxed

What type of contraction is occurring?
concentric/eccentric.

Score: ___/9

MUSCLE STABILIZATIONS

Circle the letter of the best answer to the question.

1. Which of the following muscles can stabilize the metatarsophalangeal and interphalangeal joints of toes 2 through 5?
   a. Plantaris
   b. Gastrocnemius
   c. Flexor hallucis longus
   d. Flexor digitorum longus

2. Which of the following muscles can stabilize the knee joint and the subtalar joints?
   a. Soleus
   b. Gastrocnemius
   c. Popliteus
   d. Tibialis posterior

3. Which of the following muscles stabilizes the knee joint?
   a. Popliteus
   b. Soleus
   c. Tibialis posterior
   d. Flexor digitorum longus

4. Which of the following muscles can stabilize the ankle joint, subtalar joint, and the metatarsophalangeal and interphalangeal joints of the big toe?
   a. Popliteus
   b. Soleus
   c. Flexor hallucis longus
   d. Flexor digitorum longus

Score: ___/4

YOU'VE GOT NERVE!

Write in the name of the corresponding innervation from the list provided. Choices can be used more than once.

Tibial nerve

Common fibular nerve

Deep fibular nerve

1. Gastrocnemius _____

2. Soleus _____

3. Plantaris _____

4. Tibialis posterior _____

5. Flexor digitorum longus _____

6. Flexor hallucis longus _____

7. Popliteus _____

Score: ___/7

259

ARE YOU FEELING IT? – PALPATION

Fill in the blank with the best answer to the palpation question.

1. What is the position of the knee joint when engaging and palpating the soleus?

_____

2. What is the position of the knee joint when engaging and palpating the gastrocnemius?

_____

3. Where is the distal tendon of tibialis posterior superficial and palpable?

_____

4. Where is the belly of the flexor digitorum longus superficial and palpable?

_____

5. What action do we ask the client to perform to engage and palpate the popliteus?

_____

6. Where is the popliteus most easily palpable?

_____

Score: ___/6

CLINICALLY SPEAKING

Fill in the blank with the best answer for the treatment consideration question.

1. Where did Achilles' mother hold him as she dipped him into the River Styx?

_____

2. Behind every great gastrocnemius is a great _____.

3. What muscle is sometimes thought of as the medial stirrup muscle instead of the tibialis anterior?

_____

4. What muscle is usually involved in posterior shin splints?

_____

5. What muscle has attachments into the lateral meniscus of the knee joint?

_____

Score: ___/5

Fill in the blank with the best answer to the question.

1. What are the names of the two heads of the gastrocnemius?

   _____

2. Where is the soleus most superficial?

   _____

3. What knee joint position stretches the gastrocnemius?

   _____

4. What is the insertion (distal attachment) of the triceps surae group?

   _____

5. Who are the Tom, Dick, and Harry Muscles?

   _____

   _____

6. What are the names of the three muscles/heads that comprise the triceps surae?

   _____

   _____

7. Why are the Tom, Dick, and Harry muscles grouped together?

   _____

   _____

8. Where do the Tom, Dick, and Harry muscles have superficial exposure?

   _____

9. What are the names of the four muscles located in the deep posterior compartment of the leg?

   _____

   _____

10. What are the names of the three muscles in the superficial posterior compartment of the leg?

   _____

   _____

Score: ___/10

Use the clues to complete the crossword puzzle.

ACROSS

1 Flexes and rotates the knee joint
3 Innervates all muscles of the posterior leg
7 Nickname of flexor hallucis longus
8 Superficial muscle of leg
10 Nickname of tibialis posterior

DOWN

1 Its distal tendon attaches near the Achilles tendon
2 Nickname of flexor digitorum longus
4 Shot Achilles
5 Achilles tendon
6 Popliteus _____ rotates the thigh at the knee joint
8 Stomach
9 Tom, Dick, and Harry plantarflex and _____

Score: ___/12

Fill in the blank with the best answer for the clinical case study questions.

1. A new client presents with pain and tightness in the posterior leg. During the history, you find out that she wears high-heeled shoes on a regular basis. What musculature do you suspect as being shortened and tight?

_____

_____

2. In the previous case study, what stretches do you use to help the client?

_____

_____

3. A dancer comes to you for tightness and pain in her posterior leg. Her superficial musculature feels loose. What condition is likely?

_____

_____

4. During history, a new client states that he often has posterior knee tightness and that his orthopedist told him that he has damage to his lateral meniscus. What deep muscle of the leg should be assessed and treated if tight?

_____

Score: ___/4

Section 3 tests your knowledge of the muscles covered in pages 416–430 of the *Know the Body* textbook.

KNOW YOUR MUSCLES

Fill in the blank with the name of the muscles shown.

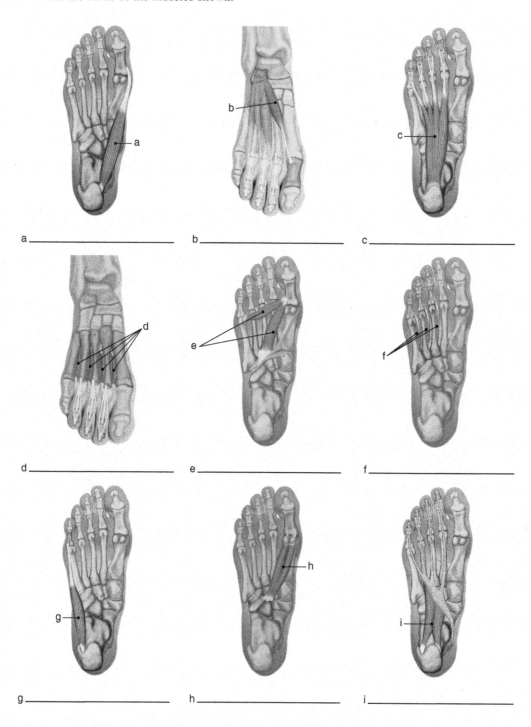

a _____

b _____

c _____

d _____

e _____

f _____

g _____

h _____

i _____

Score: ___/9

Match the muscle name from the right column to its meaning in the left column. Write your answer in the space provided. Each choice can be used only once.

Meaning

_____ 1. Located between the bones on the plantar side

_____ 2. Shorter muscle that flexes the digits

_____ 3. Square-shaped and located on the plantar side of the foot

_____ 4. Shorter muscle that extends the digits

_____ 5. Shorter muscle that flexes the big toe

_____ 6. Abducts the big toe

_____ 7. Adducts the big toe

_____ 8. Earthworm-shaped muscles of the foot

_____ 9. Flexes the little toe

_____ 10. Located between the bones on the dorsal side of the foot

_____ 11. Shorter muscle that extends the big toe

_____ 12. Abducts the little toe

Muscle name

a. Extensor digitorum brevis

b. Extensor hallucis brevis

c. Abductor hallucis

d. Abductor digiti minimi pedis

e. Flexor digitorum brevis

f. Lumbricals pedis

g. Quadratus plantae

h. Flexor hallucis brevis

i. Flexor digiti minimi pedis

j. Adductor hallucis

k. Plantar interossei

l. Dorsal interossei pedis

Score: ____/12

MATCHING ATTACHMENTS

Match each muscle from the word bank with its attachments. Write the answer in the column labeled *Muscle*. Each choice will be used only once.

Extensor digitorum brevis	Extensor hallucis brevis	Lumbricals pedis
Abductor digiti minimi pedis	Abductor hallucis	Plantar interossei
Flexor digiti minimi pedis	Flexor hallucis brevis	Quadratus plantae
Flexor digitorum brevis	Dorsal interossei pedis	Adductor hallucis

Attachments	Muscle

1. Dorsal surface of the calcaneus
   to
   Toes 2 through 4	

2. Dorsal surface of the calcaneus
   to the
   Dorsal surface of the big toe (toe 1)	

3. Tuberosity of the calcaneus
   to the
   Big toe (toe 1)	

4. Tuberosity of the calcaneus *to the* Little toe (toe 5)	
5. Tuberosity of the calcaneus *to* Toes 2 through 5	
6. The distal tendons of the flexor digitorum longus muscle *to the* Dorsal digital expansion	
7. The calcaneus *to the* Distal tendon of the flexor digitorum longus muscle	
8. Cuboid and the third cuneiform *to the* Big toe (toe 1)	
9. Fifth metatarsal *to the* Little toe (toe 5)	
10. Metatarsals *to the* Big toe (toe 1)	
11. Metatarsals *to the* Second-toe sides of the proximal phalanges of toes 3 through 5	
12. Metatarsals *to the* Sides of the phalanges (the sides away from the center of the 2nd toe)	

Score: ___/12

THE BIG PICTURE – FUNCTIONAL GROUPS

Fill in the blanks with 1) the direction of movement, 2) the body part that is moving, and 3) the joint at which movement is occurring.

1. If a muscle crosses toe joints on the plantar side, what action can it perform?

_____ of the _____.

2. If a muscle crosses toe joints on the dorsal side, what action can it perform?

_____ of the _____.

3. If a muscle crosses toe joints on the side facing the second toe, what action can it perform?

_____ of the _____.

4. If a muscle crosses toe joints on the side that faces away from the second toe, what action can it perform?

_____ of the _____.

Score: ___/4

MATCHING ACTIONS

Place the corresponding joint action letter(s) in the blank(s) next to the muscle. The number of blanks next to each muscle name indicates the number of letters that should be placed next to that muscle.

Joint Actions

a. Flexes toes 2 through 5 at the metatarsophalangeal joints

b. Flexes toes 2 through 5 at the metatarsophalangeal and proximal interphalangeal joints

c. Flexes toes 2 through 5 at the metatarsophalangeal, proximal interphalangeal and distal interphalangeal joints

d. Flexes the big toe at the metatarsophalangeal joint

e. Flexes the little toe at the metatarsophalangeal joint

f. Extends the big toe at the metatarsophalangeal joint

g. Extends toes 2 through 4 at the metatarsophalangeal, proximal interphalangeal, and distal interphalangeal joints

h. Extends toes 2 through 5 at the proximal interphalangeal and distal interphalangeal joints

i. Abducts the big toe at the metatarsophalangeal joint

j. Abducts the little toe at the metatarsophalangeal joint

k. Abducts toes 2 through 4 at the metatarsophalangeal joint

l. Adducts the big toe at the metatarsophalangeal joint

m. Adducts toes 3 through 5 at the metatarsophalangeal joint

Muscle name

1. Extensor digitorum brevis ____

2. Extensor hallucis brevis ____

3. Abductor hallucis ____

4. Abductor digiti minimi pedis ____

5. Flexor digitorum brevis ____

6. Lumbricals pedis ____ ____

7. Quadratus plantae ____

8. Flexor hallucis brevis ____

9. Flexor digiti minimi pedis ____

10. Adductor hallucis ____

11. Plantar interossei ____

12. Dorsal interossei pedis ____

Score: ___/13

THE LONG AND THE SHORT OF IT – EXERCISE 1

For each joint action given, indicate whether the muscle shortens or lengthens.

1. Lumbricals pedis: extension of toes 2 through 5 at the proximal interphalangeal and distal interphalangeal joints:

   _____

2. Quadratus plantae: flexion of toes 2 through 5 at the metatarsophalangeal, proximal interphalangeal and distal

   interphalangeal joints: _____

3. Plantar interossei: abduction of toes 3 through 5 at the metatarsophalangeal joint: _____

4. Dorsal interossei pedis: adduction of toes 2 through 4 at the metatarsophalangeal joint: _____

5. Extensor digitorum brevis: extension of toes 2 through 4 at the metatarsophalangeal, proximal interphalangeal,

   and distal interphalangeal joints: _____

Score: ___/5

Chapter **11 Muscles of the Leg and Foot**

THE LONG AND THE SHORT OF IT – EXERCISE 2

For each joint action given, fill in the blanks with a muscle that shortens and a muscle that lengthens. Please note that possible answers may be covered in another section.

1. Abduction of the toes:

   Shortens: _____ Lengthens: _____

2. Adduction of the toes:

   Shortens: _____ Lengthens: _____

3. Extension of the big toe:

   Shortens: _____ Lengthens: _____

4. Flexion of toes 2 through 5:

   Shortens: _____ Lengthens: _____

5. Flexion of the big toe:

   Shortens: _____ Lengthens: _____

Score: ___/10

MOVERS & ANTAGONISTS – EXERCISE 1

For each joint action stated, fill in the blank for a mover and antagonist of that joint action. Please choose your mover/antagonist pairs from the word bank below. Each pair can be used once and only once.

   4th Dorsal interosseus pedis/2nd Plantar interosseus

   1st Plantar interosseus/2nd Dorsal interosseus pedis

   Flexor digitorum brevis/Extensor digitorum longus

   Adductor hallucis/Abductor hallucis

1. Adducts the big toe at the metatarsophalangeal joint:

   _____

2. Flexes toes 2 through 5 at the metatarsophalangeal joints:

   _____

3. Abducts the 4th toe at the metatarsophalangeal joint:

   _____

4. Adducts the 3rd toe at the metatarsophalangeal joint:

   _____

Score: ___/4

For each joint action illustrated, the body part is being *slowly* moved in the direction indicated by the arrow. Circle whether the functional muscle group of the pair provided is contracting or relaxed. Then circle *how* the muscle group that is working is contracting (concentrically or eccentrically).

1.

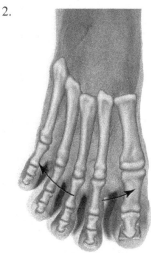

Movement:

Extension of toes at the metatarsophalangeal joints (extensors/flexors)

    Extensors: contracting/relaxed

    Flexors: contracting/relaxed

    What type of contraction is occurring? concentric/eccentric

2.

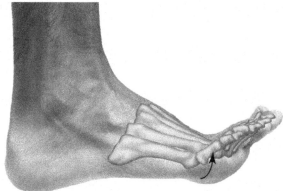

Movement:

Abduction of toes at the metatarsophalangeal joints (abductors/adductors)

    Abductors: contracting/relaxed

    Adductors: contracting/relaxed

    What type of contraction is occurring? concentric/eccentric

3.

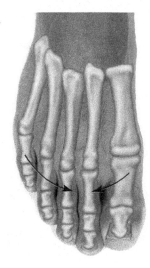

Movement:

Adduction of toes at the metatarsophalangeal joints (adductors/abductors)

    Adductors: contracting/relaxed

    Abductors: contracting/relaxed

    What type of contraction is occurring? concentric/eccentric

Score: ___/9

MUSCLE STABILIZATIONS

Circle the letter of the best answer to the question.

1. Which of the following muscles stabilizes toes 3, 4, and 5?
   a. Plantar interossei
   b. Extensor hallucis brevis
   c. Flexor digiti minimi pedis
   d. Extensor digitorum brevis

2. Which of the following muscles does NOT stabilize the little toe?
   a. Abductor digiti minimi pedis
   b. Extensor digitorum longus
   c. Dorsal interossei pedis
   d. Quadratus plantae

3. Which of the following muscles stabilizes only the metatarsophalangeal joint of the little toe?
   a. Flexor digitorum brevis
   b. Quadratus plantae
   c. Lumbricals pedis
   d. Flexor digiti minimi pedis

4. Which of the following muscles can stabilize the big toe at the metatarsophalangeal and interphalangeal joints?
   a. Abductor hallucis
   b. Flexor hallucis brevis
   c. Extensor hallucis longus
   d. Adductor hallucis

Score: ___/4

YOU'VE GOT NERVE!

Write in the name of the corresponding innervation(s) from the list provided. A choice can be used more than once.

Deep fibular nerve

Lateral plantar nerve

Medial plantar nerve

1. Extensor digitorum brevis _____

2. Extensor hallucis brevis _____

3. Abductor hallucis _____

4. Abductor digiti minimi pedis _____

5. Flexor digitorum brevis _____

6. Lumbricals pedis _____ & _____

7. Quadratus plantae _____

8. Flexor hallucis brevis _____

9. Flexor digiti minimi pedis _____

10. Adductor hallucis _____

11. Plantar interossei _____

12. Dorsal interossei pedis _____

Score: ___/12

ARE YOU FEELING IT? – PALPATION

Fill in the blank with the best answer to the palpation question.

1. Where is resistance added when engaging and palpating the extensor digitorum brevis?

_____

2. Where are the bellies of extensors digitorum and hallucis brevis palpated?

_____

3. Where do we palpate for the abductor hallucis?

_____

4. Where do we palpate for the abductor digiti minimi pedis?

_____

5. It is difficult to palpate and discern the quadratus plantae from what muscle?

_____

6. What joint of the big toe does the client flex when engaging and palpating the flexor hallucis brevis?

_____

7. Where are dorsal interossei pedis muscles palpated?

_____

Score: ___/7

CLINICALLY SPEAKING

Fill in the blank with the best answer for the treatment consideration question.

1. What intrinsic muscles attach into the plantar fascia?

_____

2. What muscle straightens out the pull of the flexor digitorum longus?

_____

3. What name is given to the adductor hallucis if it has attachments on the first metatarsal?

_____

4. What name is given to the flexor digiti minimi pedis if it has attachments on the fifth metatarsal?

_____

5. Why is intrinsic musculature of the foot so often weakened?

_____

6. Which toes have plantar interossei? Which toes have dorsal interossei pedis?

_____

Score: ___/6

MUSCLE MASH-UP

Fill in the blank with the best answer to the question.

1. What are the two heads of the adductor hallucis?

_____

2. What are the intrinsic muscles of plantar layer I?

_____

_____

3. What are the intrinsic muscles of plantar layer II?

_____

_____

4. What are the intrinsic muscles of plantar layer III?

_____

_____

5. What are the intrinsic muscles of plantar layer IV?

_____

_____

6. What are the dorsal intrinsic muscles of the foot?

_____

_____

7. Why is the word *pedis* added to the names of many intrinsic muscles of the foot?

_____

_____

8. What does interossei mean?

_____

9. To which toes does extensor digitorum brevis attach?

_____

10. The intrinsic plantar muscles of which layer all attach into the plantar fascia?

_____

_____

11. Which intrinsic plantar muscle attaches from the tendons of one muscle into the tendons of another muscle?

_____

12. Which plantar layer has two abductors and a flexor?

_____

13. Which plantar layer has two flexors and an adductor?

_____

Score: ___/13

Use the clues to complete the crossword puzzle.

ACROSS

8 Straightens out the flexor digitorum longus (two words)
9 Foot
10 Weaken intrinsic foot musculature
11 Number of named dorsal intrinsic foot muscles
12 Earthworm

DOWN

1 Fascia of foot
2 The flexor hallucis brevis has one of these bones
3 Big toe
4 Opposition would make our feet _____
5 Calcaneal attachment of plantar layer I
6 The second toe cannot do this
7 The interossei are between these

Score: ___/12

MINI CASE STUDIES

Fill in the blank with the best answer for the clinical case study questions.

1. A client presents with taut plantar fascia. What intrinsic muscles of the foot should be massaged and stretched?

_____

_____

2. A client has a collapsed arch on weight bearing. Is there benefit in massage and stretching the intrinsic muscles of the foot? Why?

_____

_____

3. What advice might be given to a client who has weak intrinsic musculature of the foot?

_____

Score: ___/3

MNEMONICS

Create your own mnemonic for the muscle group.

Lateral compartment muscles.

Fibularis Longus, Fibularis Brevis

Feet Love Fuzzy Booties!

Now make one of your own:

F _____ L _____ F _____ B _____ .

Dorsal foot muscles:

Extensor Digitorum Brevis, Extensor Hallucis Brevis

Every Day Begin Exercises Healthy Bodies!

Now make one of your own:

E _____ D _____ B _____ E _____ H _____

B _____.

Plantar layer I:

Abductor Hallucis, Abductor Digiti Minimi Pedis, Flexor Digitorum Brevis

Able Hospital Aides Diligently Make Patient's Fluffy Down Beds!

Now make one of your own:

A _____ H _____ A _____ D _____ M _____

P _____ F _____ D _____ B _____.

Plantar layer II Muscles:

Quadratus Plantae, Lumbricals Pedis

Quiet Please Loud People!

Now make one of your own:

Q _____ P _____ L _____ P _____.

Plantar layer IV muscles:

Plantar Interossei, Dorsal Interossei Pedis

Put It Down Izzie, Please!

Now make one of your own:

P _____ I _____ D _____ I _____ P _____.

CHAPTERS 9-11 SUMMARY REVIEW - MULTIPLE CHOICE

Circle the letter of the best answer to the question.

1. What muscle can be palpated between the zygomatic arch and the angle of the mandible?
   a. Medial pterygoid
   b. Lateral pterygoid
   c. Masseter
   d. Temporalis

2. What nerve innervates the Buccinator, Risorius, Nasalis, and Procerus muscles?
   a. Oculomotor (CN III)
   b. Facial (CN VII)
   c. Trochlear (CN IV)
   d. Trigeminal (CN V)

3. What nerve innervates the Temporalis, Masseter, and Medial and Lateral pterygoid muscles?
   a. Oculomotor (CN III)
   b. Facial (CN VII)
   c. Trochlear (CN IV)
   d. Trigeminal (CN V)

4. With regard to the masseter, which of the following statements is true?
   a. It is highly developed in many animals, but non-functional in humans
   b. A thick layer of fascia overlies it
   c. To engage and palpate the muscle, the client must elevate the eyebrows
   d. It is often stated to be the most powerful muscle in the human body, proportional to its size

5. Which of the following muscles can stabilize the sacrum at both the lumbosacral and the sacroiliac joints?
   a. Quadratus femoris
   b. Piriformis
   c. Gluteus medius
   d. Gluteus minimus

6. What nerve innervates the sartorius, iliacus, and pectineus muscles?
   a. Obturator
   b. Sciatic
   c. Femoral
   d. Superior gluteal

7. What muscle is superficially located in the medial thigh between the gracilis and medial hamstrings (semitendinosus and semimembranosus)?
    a. Tensor fascia latae
    b. Sartorius
    c. Adductor magnus
    d. Adductor longus

8. The gracilis is the only muscle of the adductor group to cross which of the following joints?
    a. Knee joint
    b. Hip joint
    c. Sacroiliac joint
    d. Ankle joint

9. To palpate the hamstrings proximally, what bony landmark should be located?
    a. Greater trochanter
    b. Anterior superior iliac spine
    c. Tibial tuberosity
    d. Ischial tuberosity

10. What action do all three muscles of the fibularis group perform on the foot?
    a. Plantarflexion
    b. Dorsiflexion
    c. Inversion
    d. Eversion

11. What nerve innervates the soleus, gastrocnemius, and plantaris muscles?
    a. Superficial fibular
    b. Common fibular
    c. Tibial
    d. Deep fibular

Score: ___/11

Chapter **11** **Muscles of the Leg and Foot**

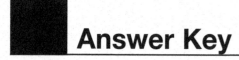

Answer Key

CHAPTER 1   BASIC KINESIOLOGY TERMINOLOGY

Major Body Parts

Coloring & Labeling

a. 1
b. 6
c. 10
d. 5
e. 2
f. 7
g. 11
h. 14
i. 8
j. 9
k. 3
l. 13
m. 4
n. 12

Matching

1. f. Arm
2. e. Forearm
3. g. Hand
4. b. Pelvis
5. a. Thigh
6. d. Leg
7. c. Foot

True or False

1. False
2. False
3. False
4. True
5. True
6. True
7. False

Fill in the Blank

1. axial body; appendicular body
2. knee joint and ankle joint
3. pelvis
4. forearm
5. leg

Multiple Choice

1. a.
2. d.
3. c.
4. c.
5. b.

Crossword Puzzle

Across

1 Pelvis
5 Appendicular
7 Leg
8 Thigh
9 Forearm
10 Arm

Down

2 Shoulder Girdle
3 Head
4 Trunk
5 Axial
6 Foot
9 Four

Anatomic Position and Location Terminology

Name the Point

1. Superior and medial
2. Distal and lateral

Matching

1. c. Posterior
2. f. Lateral
3. e. Inferior
4. h. Distal
5. a. Dorsal
6. d. Deep
7. i. Ulnar
8. g. Fibular
9. a. Dorsal
10. a. Dorsal
11. b. Caudal

True or False

1. False
2. False
3. True
4. False
5. True
6. True
7. False

Fill in the Blank

1. anatomic position
2. entire body–axial and appendicular
3. foot
4. ventral
5. proximal

Multiple Choice

1. c
2. a
3. d
4. a
5. b

Crossword Puzzle

Across	Down
2 Lateral	1 Proximal
3 Deep	4 Posterior
5 Plantar	7 Palmar
6 Superficial	8 Inferior
10 Medial	9 Anterior
11 Fibula	
12 Forward	

Planes and Axes

Name the Plane or Axis

1. Sagittal and Transverse
2. Anteroposterior and superoinferior (vertical)

Matching

Description of movement	Name of plane	Corresponding axis
Vertical: anterior to posterior	Sagittal	Mediolateral
Vertical: side to side	Frontal	Anteroposterior
Horizontal	Transverse	Superoinferior (vertical)
Oblique	Oblique	Oblique

True or False

1. False
2. True
3. False
4. True
5. True

Fill in the Blank

1. sagittal, frontal (coronal), transverse
2. axis
3. To describe the motion of a body part through space.
4. Mediolateral, anteroposterior, superoinferior (vertical)
5. axial

Multiple Choice

1. d
2. b
3. a
4. a
5. a

Crossword Puzzle

Across	Down
4 Axial	1 Vertical
6 Transverse	2 Oblique
7 Plane	3 Frontal
9 Cardinal	5 Perpendicular
10 Nonaxial	8 Sagittal
12 Mediolateral	11 Axes

Movement Terminology

Name the Motion

a. ulnar deviation (adduction) of the hand at the wrist joint
b. flexion of the leg at the knee joint
c. anterior tilt of the pelvis at the hip joints
d. dorsiflexion of the foot at the ankle joint
e. left lateral flexion of the head and neck at the spinal joints
f. flexion of the arm at the glenohumeral joint
g. extension of the trunk at the spinal joints
h. lateral rotation of the leg at the knee joint
i. abduction of the arm at the glenohumeral joint

Matching

Movement	Plane	Axis
Flexion/Extension	Sagittal	Mediolateral
Abduction/Adduction	Frontal	Anteroposterior
Right lateral flexion/Left lateral flexion	Frontal	Anteroposterior
Left rotation/Right rotation	Transverse	Vertical
Lateral rotation	Transverse	Vertical
Dorsiflexion/Plantarflexion	Sagittal	Mediolateral

True or False

1. False
2. True
3. True
4. False
5. False

Fill in the Blank

1. hyperextension
2. Forearm and foot
3. contralateral rotator
4. Cardinal plane motions
5. Opposition of the thumb

Multiple Choice

1. b
2. b
3. d
4. c
5. c

Crossword Puzzle

Across	Down
2 Medial rotation	1 Plantarflexion
3 Right rotation	5 Elevation
4 Upward	6 Abduction
8 Flexion	7 Opposition
10 Circumduction	9 Hyper
11 Extension	
12 Adduction	

The Skeletal System

Coloring & Labeling

Answers for Page Number 17
a. 11
b. 9
c. 5
d. 16
e. 1
f. 10
g. 4
h. 13
i. 7
j. 18
k. 6
l. 3
m. 19
n. 17
o. 2
p. 12
q. 22
r. 15
s. 20
t. 21
u. 14
v. 8

Answers for Page Number 18
a. 16
b. 17
c. 8
d. 21
e. 22
f. 19
g. 9
h. 2
i. 3
j. 1
k. 7
l. 18
m. 5
n. 4
o. 11
p. 14
q. 6
r. 13
s. 12
t. 15
u. 10
v. 20

Answers for Page Number 19
a. 24
b. 26
c. 9
d. 5
e. 17
f. 12
g. 6
h. 20
i. 18
j. 14
k. 22
l. 7
m. 1
n. 23
o. 21
p. 13
q. 8
r. 15
s. 25
t. 11
u. 3
v. 19
w. 16
x. 10
y. 4
z. 2

Answers for Page Number 20
a. 2
b. 21
c. 16
d. 10
e. 20
f. 5
g. 8
h. 9
i. 14
j. 17
k. 3
l. 15
m. 6
n. 23
o. 18
p. 4
q. 1
r. 19
s. 22
t. 13
u. 11
v. 24
w. 7
x. 12

Fill in the Blank

1. Femur
2. Humerus
3. Tibia and fibula
4. Radius and ulna
5. Seven
6. Scapula and clavicle
7. Five
8. Fourteen
9. Carpal
10. Tarsal
11. Ten

12. Seven
13. 206
14. Vertebrae
15. Phalanx

Know Your Bones

1. Appendicular
2. Appendicular
3. Appendicular
4. Axial
5. Axial
6. Appendicular
7. Appendicular
8. Axial
9. Appendicular
10. Axial

Crossword Puzzle

Across

4 Metacarpals
8 Femur
9 Ulna
10 Tibia
11 Tarsals

Down

1 Humerus
2 Five
3 Carpals
5 Thoracic
6 Phalanges
7 Scapula
8 Fibula

Joints

Coloring & Labeling

Answers for Page Number 23
a. 23
b. 20
c. 10
d. 16
e. 4
f. 26
g. 8
h. 1
i. 25
j. 14
k. 18
l. 15
m. 11
n. 6
o. 5
p. 22
q. 19
r. 24
s. 21
t. 7
u. 3
v. 12
w. 2
x. 13
y. 17
z. 9

Answers for Page Number 24
a. 25
b. 20
c. 16
d. 9
e. 10
f. 21
g. 18
h. 23
i. 5
j. 13
k. 15
l. 11
m. 19
n. 12
o. 7
p. 6
q. 17
r. 1
s. 3
t. 4
u. 2
v. 22
w. 14
x. 24
y. 8

Answers for Page Number 25
a. 28
b. 30
c. 4
d. 8
e. 26
f. 11
g. 22
h. 5
i. 17
j. 16
k. 18
l. 31
m. 19
n. 2
o. 13
p. 12
q. 20
r. 6
s. 14
t. 27
u. 1
v. 3
w. 21
x. 7
y. 24
z. 10
aa. 25
bb. 29
cc. 15
dd. 9
ee. 23

Answers for Page Number 26

a. 8
b. 11
c. 2
d. 7
e. 27
f. 9
g. 14
h. 10
i. 17
j. 4
k. 21
l. 16
m. 23
n. 6
o. 24
p. 19
q. 18
r. 13
s. 5
t. 3
u. 20
v. 12
w. 22
x. 26
y. 25
z. 15
aa. 1

Answers for Page Number 27

a. 7
b. 17
c. 19
d. 16
e. 4
f. 12
g. 6
h. 8
i. 2
j. 15
k. 13
l. 11
m. 10
n. 1
o. 18
p. 9
q. 14
r. 5
s. 3

Matching

1. g
2. h
3. j
4. d
5. f
6. e
7. a
8. b
9. i
10. c

True or False

1. False
2. True
3. True
4. True
5. False

Fill in the Blank

1. Two (or more) bones united by soft tissue
2. Fibrous, cartilaginous, synovial
3. Allows motion between two (or more) bones
4. Synarthrotic, amphiarthrotic, diarthrotic
5. Uniaxial, biaxial, triaxial, nonaxial

Multiple Choice

1. b
2. d
3. a
4. c
5. b

Crossword Puzzle

Across	Down
3 Biaxial	1 Carpometacarpal
6 Hinge	2 Saddle
7 Diarthrotic	4 Synovial
10 Cartilaginous	5 Fibrous
11 Pivot	8 Uniaxial
12 Triaxial	9 Nonaxial

CHAPTER 3   HOW MUSCLES FUNCTION

Coloring & Labeling

a. 1
b. 5
c. 3
d. 4
e. 2

Matching

1. c. e
2. a. f
3. b. d

Line Matching

1. Step 1
2. Step 4
3. Step 2
4. Step 3
5. Step 5

Contractions

1. Concentric
2. Relaxed
3. Eccentric
4. Relaxed
5. Isometric
6. Relaxed
7. Concentric
8. Relaxed
9. Eccentric

282

Answer Key

10. Relaxed
11. Isometric
12. Relaxed
13. Yes. When moving up away from the ground against gravity, mover muscles contracted concentrically; when slowly moving down with gravity, gravity was the mover, so the same muscles became antagonists that had to eccentrically contract to slow and guide the descent of the body part. The "other" muscle group was always relaxed.

Actions

1. Reverse
2. Standard
3. Standard
4. Reverse
5. Standard
6. Reverse
7. Reverse
8. Reverse
9. Standard
10. Standard

True or False

1. False
2. False
3. True
4. True
5. True

Fill In the Blank

1. Pulling forces
2. When the foot is planted on the ground
3. Pulling oneself up using a chin up bar, banister, handicap bar, or being helped up by someone else
4. Endomysium, perimysium, epimysium
5. Concentric
6. Longitudinal (non-pennate) and pennate
7. 1. What joint does the muscle cross? 2. Where does it cross the joint? and 3. How does it cross the joint?
8. Vertically, horizontally
9. Functional group
10. Rubber band

Multiple Choice

1. d
2. c
3. c
4. d
5. b

Crossword Puzzle

Across	Down
3 Pennate	1 Myosin
8 Insertion	2 Filament
9 Fascicle	4 Origin
11 Reverse	5 Isometric
12 Actin	6 Concentric
	7 Attempts
	10 Border

How to Palpate

Know Your Muscles

a. Deltoid
b. Flexor carpi radialis
c. Pronator teres
d. Brachialis
e. Pectoralis minor

Matching

1. h. Pronator teres
2. c. Tensor fasciae latae
3. f. Sternocleidomastoid
4. b. Brachialis
5. j. Levator scapulae
6. i. Piriformis
7. e. Rhomboids
8. d. Tibialis anterior
9. a. Psoas major
10. g. Flexor pollicis longus

True or False

1. True
2. True
3. False
4. True
5. False
6. False
7. True

Fill in the Blank

1. Know the attachments of the target muscle; know the actions of the target muscle.
2. Whenever we are contacting the client.
3. Locate and assess the target muscle.
4. (Palpating) hands
5. Palpate slowly and have the client breathe

Multiple Choice

General Palpation

1. d
2. c
3. c
4. d
5. a
6. c
7. b
8. a
9. b
10. c

Multiple Choice

Isolated Contraction

1. c
2. b
3. a
4. c
5. c

Multiple Choice

Resistance

1. a
2. b
3. c
4. d
5. b

Crossword Puzzle

Across

2 Palpation
5 Coupled
11 Inhibition
12 Assess
14 Alternately

Down

1 Baby
3 Appropriate
4 Ticklish
6 Critically
7 Resistance
8 Mindful Touch
9 Literacy
10 Isolated
13 Strum

CHAPTER 5   BONY PALPATION

Upper Extremity

Coloring & Labeling

Answers for Page Number 44–Anteromedial View

a. 5
b. 4
c. 1
d. 6
e. 3
f. 2

Answers for Page Number 44–Posterolateral View

a. 8
b. 3
c. 4
d. 7
e. 5
f. 9
g. 6
h. 2
i. 1

Answers for Page Number 44–Lateral View

a. 5
b. 4
c. 3
d. 6
e. 2
f. 1

Answers for Page Number 45–Anterior (Palmar) View

a. 4
b. 5
c. 2
d. 3
e. 1
f. 6

Answers for Page Number 45–Inferolateral View

a. 10
b. 2

c. 9
d. 7
e. 1
f. 4
g. 5
h. 3
i. 6
j. 8

Answers for Page Number 45–Lateral View

a. 4
b. 2
c. 3
d. 5
e. 7
f. 1
g. 6

Answers for Page Number 46–Superolateral View

a. 11
b. 10
c. 4
d. 3
e. 7
f. 2
g. 6
h. 5
i. 1
j. 9
k. 8

Answers for Page Number 46–Posterolateral View

a. 5
b. 2
c. 3
d. 6
e. 4
f. 1

Answers for Page Number 46–Oblique View

a. 7
b. 5
c. 2
d. 3
e. 1
f. 4
g. 6

Answers for Page Number 47–Anterolateral View

a. 7
b. 1
c. 6
d. 4
e. 2
f. 9
g. 8
h. 3
i. 5

Answers for Page Number 47–Medial View

a. 2
b. 5
c. 3
d. 6

e. 1
f. 9
g. 7
h. 8
i. 4

Answers for Page Number 47–Plantar View

a. 4
b. 5
c. 3
d. 2
e. 6
f. 1

Know Your Bones

1. Acromion process of the scapula
2. Inferior angle of the scapula
3. Clavicle
4. Medial and lateral epicondyles of the humerus
5. Dorsal tubercle (Lister's tubercle)
6. Radial head
7. Spine of the scapula
8. Coracoid process of the scapula

True or False

1. False
2. False
3. True
4. True

Fill in the Blank

1. Coracoid process of the scapula
2. Inferior angle
3. Lesser tubercle
4. Radial head

Multiple Choice

1. b. Hamate
2. c. The medial clavicle is convex; the lateral clavicle is concave
3. b. Laterally
4. d. Greater and lesser tubercles of humerus

Crossword Puzzle

Across	Down
3 Bicipital	1 Dorsal
6 Pisiform	2 Ulnar Nerve
8 Acromion	4 Coracoid
11 Lateral	5 Spine
12 Triceps	7 Hook
	9 Styloid
	10 Head

Axial Body

Know Your Bones

1. Body of the mandible
2. SPs
3. EOP
4. Xiphoid process of the sternum
5. TPs

6. Hyoid bone
7. Articular process
8. Zygomatic bone

True or False

1. False
2. True
3. True
4. True

Fill in the Blank

1. Articular pillar-/-cervical pillar
2. Carotid tubercle
3. C2 (axis) and C7
4. Take in a deep breath

Multiple Choice

1. a. Laminar groove
2. a. 1st
3. d. Facet
4. d. Anterior

Crossword Puzzle

Across	Down
3 Jugular	1 Fourteen
4 Hyoid	2 Bifid
6 Cheek	5 Intercostal
9 Transverse	7 Atlas
10 Tubercle	8 Facets
11 Laminar	10 TMJ

Lower Extremity

Know Your Bones

1. Calcaneal tuberosity
2. Tibial tuberosity
3. Navicular tuberosity
4. ASIS
5. Ischial tuberosity
6. Lateral malleolus of the fibula
7. PSIS
8. Greater trochanter of femur

True or False

1. False
2. True
3. True
4. True

Fill in the Blank

1. Anterior superior iliac spine
2. Medial malleolus
3. Navicular tuberosity
4. Fibular head

Multiple Choice

1. d. Superior to inferior
2. d. C2 spinous process
3. a. Anterolateral
4. b. Sustentaculum tali

285

Crossword Puzzle

Across

2 Ulnar
6 Pubic
8 Gluteal
10 Lesser
11 Sesamoid
12 Head

Down

1 Talus
3 Malleolus
4 Lateral
5 Dimple
7 Styloid
9 Cuboid

Chapters 1—5 Summary Review - Multiple Choice

1. c. Sagittal
2. d. Both b and c
3. b. Concentric
4. d. Fascicle
5. d. All of the above
6. a. Add resistance
7. b. Reciprocal inhibition
8. d. Have the client place a hand over their palpating hand
9. a. Pisiform
10. c. Posterior superior iliac spine

CHAPTER 6   MUSCLES OF THE SHOULDER GIRDLE AND ARM

Coloring & Labeling

Answers for Page Number 64

a. 1
b. 7
c. 9
d. 3
e. 2
f. 5
g. 6
h. 13
i. 14
j. 4
k. 8
l. 10
m. 11
n. 12

Answers for Page Number 65

a. 12
b. 1
c. 16
d. 4
e. 13
f. 2
g. 11
h. 14
i. 5
j. 10
k. 6
l. 8
m. 3
n. 7
o. 15
p. 9
q. 17

Answers for Page Number 66

a. 6
b. 9
c. 3
d. 4
e. 2
f. 1
g. 8
h. 5
i. 7
j. 10

Section 1

Know Your Muscles

a. Serratus anterior
b. Latissimus Dorsi
c. Subclavius
d. Trapezius
e. Levator scapulae
f. Rhomboid major
g. Rhomboid minor
h. Teres major
i. Pectoralis major
j. Pectoralis minor

What's in a Name?

1. g. Trapezius
2. d. Rhomboid major
3. j. Rhomboid minor
4. b. Levator scapulae
5. f. Serratus anterior
6. e. Pectoralis major
7. a. Pectoralis minor
8. i. Subclavius
9. h. Latissimus dorsi
10. c. Teres major

Matching Attachments

1. Trapezius
2. Rhomboids
3. Levator scapulae
4. Serratus anterior
5. Pectoralis major
6. Pectoralis minor
7. Subclavius
8. Latissimus dorsi
9. Teres major

The Big Picture – Functional Groups

1. Elevation, scapula, scapulocostal
2. Depression, scapula, scapulocostal
3. Protraction, scapula, scapulocostal
4. Retraction, scapula, scapulocostal
5. Flexion, arm, glenohumeral
6. Extension, arm, glenohumeral
7. Adduction, arm, glenohumeral
8. Medial rotation, arm, glenohumeral

Matching Actions

1. a, c, e, q, s, u
2. c
3. b, e
4. a, c, f
5. a, f, p, r, t
6. d, e
7. i, k, g, h, d
8. b, d, f
9. m, n
10. h, j, k
11. h, j, k

The Long and the Short of It – Exercise 1

1. Lengthens
2. Lengthens
3. Shortens
4. Shortens
5. Shortens

The Long and the Short of It – Exercise 2

1. Shortens: serratus anterior, pectoralis minor; Lengthens: upper trapezius, middle trapezius, rhomboids
2. Shortens: upper trapezius, middle trapezius, rhomboids; Lengthens: serratus anterior, pectoralis minor
3. Shortens: upper trapezius, levator scapulae; Lengthens: lower trapezius, pectoralis minor
4. Shortens: rhomboids, levator scapulae, pectoralis minor, deltoid; Lengthens: upper trapezius, lower trapezius, serratus anterior
5. Shortens: Pectoralis major, supraspinatus, anterior deltoid, coracobrachialis, biceps brachii; Lengthens: pectoralis major, latissimus dorsi, teres major, posterior deltoid, triceps brachii

Movers & Antagonists – Exercise 1

1. Serratus anterior/Rhomboids
2. Teres major/Pectoralis major
3. Upper trapezius/Lower trapezius
4. Upper trapezius/Pectoralis minor

Movers & Antagonists – Exercise 2

1. Flexors: contracting; Extensors: relaxed; Type of contraction: concentric
2. Flexors: contracting; Extensors: relaxed; Type of contraction: eccentric
3. Elevators: contracting; Depressors: relaxed; Type of contraction: concentric
4. Elevators: contracting; Depressors: relaxed; Type of contraction: eccentric

Muscle Stabilizations

1. d. All of the above
2. c. Levator scapulae
3. d. Subclavius
4. b. Teres major

You've got Nerve!

1. Spinal accessory nerve
2. Dorsal scapular nerve
3. Long thoracic nerve
4. Dorsal scapular nerve
5. Medial and lateral pectoral nerves
6. Thoracodorsal nerve

Are You Feeling It? – Palpation

1. Rhomboids, levator scapulae, pectoralis minor
2. Serratus anterior
3. Levator scapulae, splenius capitis, scalenes, omohyoid
4. Subclavius
5. Pectoralis minor
6. Trapezius

Clinically Speaking

1. Trapezius
2. Rounded/slumped shoulders (protracted scapulae)
3. Levator scapulae
4. Serratus anterior
5. Pectoralis minor

Muscle Mash-Up

1. Pectoralis minor
2. Trapezius
3. Rhomboids, levator scapulae, serratus anterior
4. Trapezius
5. Trapezius (upper and lower) and serratus anterior
6. Trapezius
7. Rhomboids
8. Serratus anterior
9. Levator scapulae
10. Teres major
11. Pectoralis major
12. Subclavius
13. Latissimus dorsi
14. Latissimus dorsi

Crossword Puzzle

Across

3 C7
6 Anterior
9 Armpit
11 Key
13 Serratus anterior
15 Middle
16 Scapula
18 CNXI
21 Bicipital
22 Extension

Down

1 Minor
2 Major
3 Clavicular
4 Rhomboids
5 Teres major
7 Outlet
8 Antagonistic
10 Trapezius
12 Elevation
14 Deep
17 Left
19 Anterior
20 Nine

Mini Case Studies

1. Pectoralis minor
2. Upper trapezius and levator scapulae
3. Subclavius, pectoralis minor, pectoralis major
4. Latissimus dorsi

Know Your Muscles

a. Deltoid
b. Biceps brachii
c. Supraspinatus
d. Teres minor
e. Infraspinatus
f. Triceps brachii
g. Coracobrachialis
h. Subscapularis
i. Brachialis

What's in a Name?

1. e. Supraspinatus
2. c. Infraspinatus
3. b. Teres minor
4. j. Subscapularis
5. a. Deltoid
6. h. Coracobrachialis
7. i. Biceps brachii
8. f. Brachialis
9. g. Triceps brachii
10. d. Anconeus

Matching Attachments

1. Supraspinatus
2. Infraspinatus
3. Teres minor
4. Subscapularis
5. Deltoid
6. Coracobrachialis
7. Biceps brachii
8. Brachialis
9. Triceps brachii
10. Anconeus

The Big Picture – Functional Groups

1. Flexion, arm, glenohumeral
2. Extension, arm, glenohumeral
3. Adduction, arm, glenohumeral
4. Abduction, arm, glenohumeral
5. Lateral rotation, arm, glenohumeral
6. Medial rotation, arm, glenohumeral
7. Flexion, forearm, elbow
8. Extension, forearm, elbow
9. Reverse action

Matching Actions

1. a, c
2. e
3. e
4. f
5. c, i
6. a, f, g, c
7. b, e, h, c
8. a, d
9. a, j, l

10. j
11. b, k
12. k

The Long and the Short of It – Exercise 1

1. Shortens
2. Lengthens
3. Lengthens
4. Shortens
5. Lengthens

The Long and the Short of It – Exercise 2

1. Shortens: supraspinatus, anterior deltoid, coracobrachialis, biceps brachii; Lengthens: posterior deltoid, triceps brachii, latissimus dorsi, teres major
2. Shortens: posterior deltoid, triceps brachii, latissimus dorsi, teres major; Lengthens: supraspinatus, anterior deltoid, coracobrachialis, biceps brachii
3. Shortens: infraspinatus, teres minor, posterior deltoid; Lengthens: subscapularis, anterior deltoid, pectoralis major, latissimus dorsi, teres major
4. Shortens: coracobrachialis, pectoralis major; Lengthens: supraspinatus, entire deltoid
5. Shortens: biceps brachii, brachialis; Lengthens: triceps brachii, anconeus

Movers & Antagonists – Exercise 1

1. Infraspinatus/Subscapularis
2. Supraspinatus/Coracobrachialis
3. Triceps brachii/Brachialis
4. Anterior deltoid/Posterior deltoid

Movers & Antagonists – Exercise 2

1. Abductors: contracting; Adductors: relaxed; Type of contraction: concentric
2. Abductors: contracting; Adductors: relaxed; Type of contraction: eccentric
3. Lateral rotators: contracting: Medial rotators: relaxed; Type of contraction: concentric
4. Lateral rotators: relaxed; Medial rotators: contracting; Type of contraction: concentric

Muscle Stabilizations

1. d. All of the above
2. a. Biceps brachii
3. d. Triceps brachii
4. c. Anconeus

You've Got Nerve!

1. Axillary nerve
2. Suprascapular nerve
3. Musculocutaneous nerve
4. Radial nerve
5. Musculocutaneous nerve
6. Upper and lower subscapular nerves

Are you Feeling it? – Palpation

1. Distal arm (not the forearm)
2. Deltoid
3. Triceps brachii (long head), infraspinatus, teres minor and teres major
4. Subscapularis
5. Anterior fibers
6. Full pronation

Clinically Speaking

1. Supraspinatus
2. Deltoid or supraspinatus
3. Ulnar and median nerves and brachial artery
4. Long head
5. Triceps brachii

Muscle Mash-Up

1. Anterior, middle, and posterior
2. Brachialis
3. Laterally rotate and abduct the arm
4. No
5. Infraspinatus and teres minor
6. Teres minor
7. Deltoid (posterior fibers)
8. Trapezius (upper)
9. False
10. True
11. Musculocutaneous
12. Biceps brachii (short head), coracobrachialis, and pectoralis minor
13. Triceps brachii
14. Infraspinatus and teres minor
15. Deltoid

Crossword Puzzle

Across	Down
2 Anconeus	1 Subacromial
4 Brachialis	3 Subscapularis
10 Supraspinatus	5 Long
12 Musculocutaneous	6 Triangle
13 Infraspinatus	7 Triceps
14 Stabilization	8 Tubercle
16 Three	9 Biceps
17 Deltoid	11 Downward
18 Armpit	14 Short
19 Radial	15 Lateral

Mini Case Studies

1. Brachialis
2. Deltoid (especially middle fibers) and supraspinatus
3. Subscapularis
4. Deltoid

CHAPTER 7   MUSCLES OF THE FOREARM AND HAND

Coloring & Labeling

Answers for Page Number 89

a. 14
b. 2
c. 6
d. 17
e. 18
f. 3
g. 10
h. 7
i. 8
j. 19
k. 16
l. 13
m. 9
n. 1
o. 11
p. 12
q. 15
r. 4
s. 5

Answers for Page Number 90

a. 8
b. 1
c. 7
d. 16
e. 11
f. 3
g. 14
h. 10
i. 4
j. 17
k. 15
l. 13
m. 9
n. 2
o. 6
p. 12
q. 5

Answers for Page Number 91

a. 6
b. 5
c. 12
d. 17
e. 10
f. 7
g. 3
h. 15
i. 13
j. 11
k. 1
l. 2
m. 8
n. 16
o. 14
p. 9
q. 4

Answers for Page Number 92
a. 15
b. 3
c. 10
d. 5
e. 14
f. 8
g. 7
h. 2
i. 9
j. 11
k. 6
l. 4
m. 12
n. 13
o. 1

Answers for Page Number 93
a. 18
b. 8
c. 1
d. 9
e. 24
f. 6
g. 23
h. 12
i. 10
j. 15
k. 5
l. 20
m. 21
n. 2
o. 4
p. 22
q. 16
r. 17
s. 11
t. 3
u. 7
v. 19
w. 13
x. 25
y. 14

Section 1

Know Your Muscles

a. Brachioradialis
b. Flexor digitorum superficialis
c. Flexor carpi radialis
d. Palmaris longus
e. Flexor carpi ulnaris
f. Flexor pollicis longus
g. Flexor digitorum profundus
h. Pronator teres
i. Pronator quadratus

What's in a Name?

1. h. Flexor carpi ulnaris
2. g. Pronator quadratus

3. c. Flexor pollicis longus
4. d. Flexor carpi radialis
5. a. Flexor digitorum superficialis
6. b. Brachioradialis
7. f. Pronator teres
8. e. Flexor digitorum profundus
9. i. Palmaris longus

Matching Attachments

1. Flexor carpi radialis
2. Palmaris longus
3. Flexor carpi ulnaris
4. Pronator teres
5. Pronator quadrates
6. Brachioradialis
7. Flexor digitorum superficialis
8. Flexor digitorum profundus
9. Flexor pollicis longus

The Big Picture – Functional Groups

1. Flexion, hand, wrist
2. Extension, hand, wrist
3. Radial deviation (abduction), hand, wrist
4. Ulnar deviation (adduction), hand, wrist
5. Flexion, fingers 2 through 5, metacarpophalangeal and/or proximal and distal interphalangeal
6. Extension, fingers 2 through 5, metacarpophalangeal and/or proximal and distal interphalangeal
7. Pronation, forearm, radioulnar
8. Supination, forearm, radioulnar
9. Flexion, forearm, elbow
10. Extension, forearm, elbow
11. Reverse actions

Matching Actions

1. d, e
2. d
3. d, f
4. a, b
5. b
6. a, b, c
7. d, g
8. d, g
9. d, h

The Long and the Short of It – Exercise 1

1. Shortens
2. Lengthens
3. Lengthens
4. Lengthens
5. Shortens

The Long and the Short of It – Exercise 2

1. Shortens: flexor carpi radialis, palmaris longus, flexor carpi ulnaris, flexor digitorum superficialis, flexor digitorum profundus, flexor pollicis longus; Lengthens: extensor carpi radialis longus, extensor carpi radialis brevis, extensor carpi ulnaris, extensor digitorum, extensor digiti minimi

2. Shortens: extensor carpi radialis longus, extensor carpi radialis brevis, extensor carpi ulnaris, extensor digitorum, extensor digiti minimi; Lengthens: flexor carpi radialis, palmaris longus, flexor carpi ulnaris, flexor digitorum superficialis, flexor digitorum profundus, flexor pollicis longus
3. Shortens: flexor carpi radialis; Lengthens: flexor carpi ulnaris
4. Shortens: flexor digitorum superficialis, flexor digitorum profundus; Lengthens: extensor digitorum, extensor digitiminimi
5. Shortens: pronator teres, pronator quadrates, brachioradialis; Lengthens: brachioradialis, supinator

Movers & Antagonists – Exercise 1
1. Flexor carpi radialis/Flexor carpi ulnaris
2. Pronator teres/Brachioradialis

Movers & Antagonists – Exercise 2
1. Flexors: contracting; Extensors: relaxed; Type of contraction: concentric
2. Flexors: contracting; Extensors: relaxed; Type of contraction: eccentric
3. Pronators: contracting; Supinators: relaxed; Type of contraction: concentric

Muscle Stabilizations
1. c. Palmaris longus
2. d. All of the above
3. a. Pronator teres
4. b. Flexor pollicis longus

You've Got Nerve!
1. Median nerve
2. Radial nerve
3. Ulnar nerve
4. Median nerve
5. Median nerve
6. Median nerve

Are You Feeling It? – Palpation
1. On the distal forearm, not the hand
2. Brachioradialis and pronator teres
3. Flexion of the hand at the wrist joint
4. Interphalangeal
5. Flexor digitorum profundus

Clinically Speaking
1. Golfer's elbow (medial epicondylitis/epicondylosis)
2. Median
3. Brachialis, biceps brachii, brachioradialis
4. Flexor pollicis longus
5. Flexors digitorum superficialis and profundus, flexor pollicis longus

Muscle Mash-Up
1. Flexor carpi radialis, palmaris longus, flexor carpi ulnaris
2. Medial epicondyle of the humerus
3. Lateral epicondyle of the humerus
4. Flexor digitorum superficialis
5. Flexor carpi radialis
6. Flexor pollicis longus

7. Brachioradialis
8. Lateral epicondylitis or lateral epicondylosis
9. Flexor carpi radialis
10. Flexor carpi ulnaris
11. Median
12. Flexor digitorum superficialis and flexor digitorum profundus
13. Medial epicondyle of the humerus via the common flexor tendon
14. Brachioradialis and extensor carpi radialis longus
15. Extensor carpi radialis brevis

Crossword Puzzle

Across	Down
4 Median	1 Radial
5 Deep	2 Humeral
7 Teres	3 Forearm
9 Quadratus	6 Pollicis
11 Radial	8 Ulnar
12 Digitorum	10 Tennis Elbow
14 Four	13 Intrinsic
15 Hitchhiker	14 FDP
16 Extrinsic	17 Carpi
18 Five	19 Heads
21 Extension	20 ECRL
22 Brachioradialis	

Mini Case Studies
1. Muscles of the common flexor tendon (wrist flexor group, pronator teres, and flexor digitorum superficialis)
2. Flexors digitorum superficialis and profundus and flexor pollicis longus
3. Pronator teres
4. Flexor pollicis longus

Section 2

Know Your Muscles
a. Supinator
b. Abductor pollicis longus
c. Extensor pollicis brevis
d. Extensor pollicis longus
e. Extensor indicis
f. Extensor carpi radialis longus
g. Extensor carpi radialis brevis
h. Extensor carpi ulnaris
i. Extensor digitorum
j. Externsor digiti minimi

What's in a Name?
1. b. Extensor pollicis longus
2. i. Extensor pollicis brevis
3. h. Extensor carpi ulnaris
4. c. Extensor digitorum
5. g. Extensor carpi radialis longus
6. f. Extensor indicis
7. a. Abductor pollicis longus
8. j. Supinator
9. d. Extensor digiti minimi
10. e. Extensor carpi radialis brevis

Matching Attachments

1. Extensor carpi radialis longus
2. Extensor carpi radialis brevis
3. Extensor carpi ulnaris
4. Extensor digitorum
5. Extensor digiti minimi
6. Supinator
7. Abductor pollicis longus
8. Extensor pollicis brevis
9. Extensor pollicis longus
10. Extensor indicis

The Big Picture – Functional Groups

1. Flexion, hand, wrist
2. Extension, hand, wrist
3. Radial deviation (abduction), hand, wrist
4. Ulnar deviation (adduction), hand, wrist
5. Extension, fingers 2 through 5, metacarpophalangeal
6. Supination, forearm, radioulnar
7. Abduction, thumb, carpometacarpal
8. Extension, thumb, carpometacarpal

Matching Actions

1. b, c
2. b, c
3. b, d
4. b, e
5. b, e
6. a
7. f, g
8. f, g
9. f
10. e

The Long and the Short of It – Exercise 1

1. Lengthens
2. Shortens
3. Lengthens
4. Lengthens
5. Shortens

The Long and the Short of It – Exercise 2

1. Shortens: flexor carpi radialis, palmaris longus, flexor carpi ulnaris, flexor digitorum superficialis, flexor digitorum profundus, flexor pollicis longus; Lengthens: extensor carpi radialis longus, extensor carpi radialis brevis, extensor carpi ulnaris, extensor digitorum, extensor digiti minimi
2. Shortens: extensor carpi radialis longus, extensor carpi radialis brevis, extensor carpi ulnaris, extensor digitorum, extensor digiti minimi; Lengthens: flexor carpi radialis, palmaris longus, flexor carpi ulnaris, flexor digitorum superficialis, flexor digitorum profundus, flexor pollicis longus
3. Shortens: extensor carpi radialis longus, extensor carpi radialis brevis, flexor carpi radialis; Lengthens: extensor carpi ulnaris, flexor carpi ulnaris
4. Shortens: extensor carpi ulnaris, flexor carpi ulnaris; Lengthens: extensor carpi radialis longus, extensor carpi radialis brevis, flexor carpi radialis

5. Shortens: pronator teres, pronator quadrates, brachioradialis; Lengthens: supinator, brachioradialis

Movers & Antagonists – Exercise 1

1. Extensor digitorum/Flexor digitorum superficialis
2. Supinator/Pronator quadratus
3. Extensor carpi ulnaris/Extensor carpi radialis longus
4. Extensor carpi radialis brevis/Flexor carpi ulnaris
5. Flexor pollicis longus/Extensor pollicis brevis

Movers & Antagonists – Exercise 2

1. Extensors: relaxed; Flexors: contracting; Type of contraction: eccentric
2. Flexors: contracting; Extensors: relaxed; Type of contraction: concentric
3. Pronators: relaxed; Supinators: contracting; Type of contraction: concentric

Muscle Stabilizations

1. d. All of the above
2. d. All of the above
3. b. Supinator
4. a. Extensor digitorum

You've Got Nerve!

1. Radial nerve
2. Radial nerve
3. Radial nerve
4. Radial nerve
5. Radial nerve
6. Radial nerve

Are You Feeling It? – Palpation

1. Supinator
2. Extensor carpi ulnaris
3. Radial deviation of the hand at the wrist joint
4. On the hand, proximal to the fingers
5. Extensor digitorum

Clinically Speaking

1. Tennis elbow (lateral epicondylitis/epicondylosis)
2. Extensor carpi radialis brevis
3. Radial
4. Abductor pollicis longus and extensor pollicis brevis
5. Extensor carpi ulnaris and flexor digitorum profundus

Muscle Mash-Up

1. Extensor carpi radialis longus, extensor carpi radialis brevis, extensor carpi ulnaris
2. Lateral epicondyle of the humerus
3. Medial epicondyle of the humerus
4. They both do ulnar deviation of the hand at the wrist joint
5. The flexor carpi ulnaris flexes the hand; the extensor carpi ulnaris extends the hand
6. Abductor pollicis longus, extensor pollicis brevis, extensor pollicis longus
7. Index (#2) and little (#5) fingers
8. Tennis elbow
9. Brachioradialis and extensor carpi radialis longus

10. Scaphoid
11. Radial styloid
12. Extensor digitorum
13. Abductor pollicis longus and extensor pollicis brevis
14. Abductor pollicis longus and extensor pollicis brevis
15. Supinator

Mini Case Studies

1. Muscles of the common extensor tendon (extensor carpi radialis brevis, extensors digitorum and digiti minimi, extensor carpi ulnaris)
2. Abductor pollicis longus and extensor pollicis brevis
3. De Quervain's disease
4. Extensor carpi radialis brevis

Crossword Puzzle

Across

3 Forearm
7 Ulna
8 Four
10 Extensor
12 Tenosynovitis
14 EDM
17 Ulnar Deviation
20 Pollicis
21 FCU
22 Medial

Down

1 Pronator Teres
2 Radial
4 Ulnaris
5 Little Finger
6 Brachioradialis
9 ECRB
11 Five
13 Extends
15 Extrinsic
16 Supinator
18 Digitorum
19 Indicis

Section 3

Know Your Muscles

a. Palmar interossei
b. Abductor digiti minimi manus
c. Flexor digiti minimi manus
d. Lumbricals manus
e. Opponens pollicis
f. Opponens digiti minimi
g. Dorsal interossei manus
h. Abductor pollicis brevis
i. Adductor pollicis

What's in a Name?

1. j. Opponens digiti minimi
2. a. Flexor pollicis brevis
3. b. Flexor digiti minimi manus
4. f. Palmar interossei
5. c. Adductor pollicis
6. h. Palmaris brevis
7. k. Abductor pollicis brevis
8. d. Dorsal interossei manus
9. e. Lumbricals manus
10. g. Opponens pollicis
11. i. Abductor digiti minimi manus

Matching Attachments

1. Abductor pollicis brevis
2. Flexor pollicis brevis
3. Opponens pollicis
4. Abductor digiti minimi manus

5. Flexor digiti minimi manus
6. Opponens digiti minimi
7. Palmaris brevis
8. Adductor pollicis
9. Lumbricals manus
10. Palmar interossei
11. Dorsal interossei manus

The Big Picture – Functional Groups

1. Flexion, fingers two through five, carpometacarpal
2. Extension, fingers two through five, carpometacarpal
3. Adduction, finger, carpometacarpal
4. Abduction, finger, carpometacarpal
5. Abduction, thumb, carpometacarpal
6. Adduction, thumb, carpometacarpal
7. Extension, thumb, carpometacarpal
8. Flexion, thumb, carpometacarpal

Matching Actions

1. g
2. f
3. i
4. d
5. b
6. j
7. k
8. h
9. a
10. e
11. c

The Long and the Short of It – Exercise 1

1. Shortens
2. Lengthens
3. Lengthens
4. Shortens
5. Lengthens

The Long and the Short of It – Exercise 2

1. Shortens: adductor pollicis; Lengthens: abductor pollicis brevis
2. Shortens: abductor pollicis brevis; Lengthens: adductor pollicis
3. Shortens: palmar interossei; Lengthens: abductor digiti minimi manus
4. Shortens: abductor digiti minimi manus; Lengthens: palmar interossei
5. Shortens: extensor digitorum, extensor digiti minimi; Lengthens: flexor digiti minimi manus, lumbricals manus

Movers & Antagonists – Exercise 1

1. Palmar interossei/Dorsal interossei manus
2. Adductor pollicis/Abductor pollicis brevis
3. Flexor pollicis brevis/Extensor pollicis longus
4. Extensor digitorum/Flexor digitorum profundus

Muscle Stabilizations

1. d. All of the above
2. d. Abductor digiti minimi manus
3. b. Lumbricals manus

293

You've Got Nerve!

1. Median nerve
2. Median nerve, Ulnar nerve
3. Ulnar nerve
4. Ulnar nerve
5. Ulnar nerve
6. Median nerve, Ulnar nerve

Are You Feeling It? – Palpation

1. Thumb web of the hand
2. Opponens pollicis
3. Flexor pollicis brevis
4. Palmar interossei
5. Abductor digiti minimi manus

Clinically Speaking

1. Texting thumb
2. Basilar arthritis
3. Abductor digiti minimi manus
4. Adductor pollicis or flexor pollicis brevis
5. First

Muscle Mash-Up

1. Abductor pollicis brevis, flexor pollicis brevis, opponens pollicis
2. Abductor digiti minimi manus, flexor digiti minimi manus, opponens digiti minimi
3. Adductor pollicis, lumbricals manus, palmar interossei, dorsal interossei manus
4. Abductor pollicis brevis
5. Because this muscle is shorter than the flexor pollicis longus
6. Flexor retinaculum
7. Opponens pollicis
8. Opponens digiti minimi
9. Because there is an abductor digiti minimi pedis in the foot
10. Abductor digiti minimi manus
11. Palmaris brevis
12. Dorsal interossei manus
13. Lumbricals manus
14. Middle
15. Little

Crossword Puzzle

Across

3 Oblique
6 Ulnar
8 Middle
9 Interossei
12 Intrinsic
16 Adductor
18 Basilar
19 Median
20 Apes

Down

1 Four
2 Lumbricals
4 Anterolateral
5 Pollicis
7 Little
10 Sesamoid
11 Trapezium
13 Texting
14 Indicis
15 Three
17 Hamate

Mini Case Studies

1. Adductor pollicis and first dorsal interosseus
2. Basilar arthritis

3. Flexor pollicis longus, thenar eminence group (abductor and flexor pollicis brevis, opponens pollicis), thumb muscles of deep distal four group (abductor pollicis longus, extensors pollicis brevis and longus)
4. Hypothenar

CHAPTER 8   MUSCLES OF THE SPINE AND RIBCAGE

Coloring & Labeling

Answers for Page Number 126

a. 8
b. 1
c. 6
d. 2
e. 7
f. 10
g. 20
h. 13
i. 19
j. 21
k. 3
l. 18
m. 4
n. 12
o. 11
p. 15
q. 16
r. 14
s. 17
t. 9
u. 5

Answers for Page Number 127

a. 3
b. 4
c. 2
d. 10
e. 7
f. 1
g. 9
h. 11
i. 6
j. 8
k. 5

Answers for Page Number 128

a. 2
b. 8
c. 7
d. 9
e. 3
f. 6
g. 10
h. 4
i. 5
j. 1

Answers for Page Number 128

a. 2
b. 8
c. 6
d. 9
e. 3
f. 7
g. 4
h. 5
i. 1
j. 10

Answers for Page Number 129

a. 9
b. 10
c. 1
d. 5
e. 7
f. 2
g. 8
h. 4
i. 3
j. 6
k. 11

Section 1

Know Your Muscles

a. Serratus posterior superior
b. Intertransversarii
c. Erector spinae group
d. Quadratus lumborum
e. Semispinalis
f. Multifudus
g. Rotatores
h. Interspinales
i. Serratus posterior inferior

What's in a Name?

1. d. Quadratus lumborum
2. b. Serratus posterior superior
3. f. Intertransversarii
4. c. Serratus posterior inferior
5. g. Erector spinae
6. a. Transversospinalis
7. e. Interspinales

Matching Attachments

1. Erector spinae
2. Transversospinalis
3. Interspinales
4. Intertransversarii
5. Serratus posterior superior
6. Serratus posterior inferior
7. Quadratus lumborum

The Big Picture – Functional Groups

1. Extension, trunk, spinal
2. Flexion, trunk, spinal
3. Lateral flexion, trunk, spinal
4. Elevation, pelvis, lumbosacral
5. Elevation, ribs, sternocostal and costospinal
6. Depression, ribs, sternocostal and costospinal
7. Extension of the lower spine relative to the upper spine

Matching Actions

1. c, f, h
2. c, f, g, h
3. b
4. e
5. i
6. j
7. a, d, h, k, l

The Long and the Short of It – Exercise 1

1. Lengthens
2. Shortens
3. Shortens
4. Lengthens
5. Lengthens

The Long and the Short of It – Exercise 2

1. Shortens: erector spinae, transversospinalis, interspinales, quadratus lumborum; Lengthens: rectus abdominis, internal abdominal obliques, external abdominal obliques
2. Shortens: quadratus lumborum, erector spinae, transversospinalis; Lengthens: rectus abdominis, internal abdominal obliques, external abdominal obliques
3. Shortens: rectus abdominis, internal abdominal obliques, external abdominal obliques; Lengthens: quadratus lumborum, erector spinae, transversospinalis
4. Shortens: internal intercostals, subcostales, transversus thoracis, serratus posterior inferior, quadratus lumborum; Lengthens: external intercostals, levatores costarum, serratus posterior superior
5. Shortens: anterior scalene, middle scalene, sternohyoid, sternothyroid, thyrohyoid, omohyoid, longus colli, sternocleidomastoid; Lengthens: erector spinae, transversospinalis, interspinales, splenius cervicis, splenius capitis, sternocleidomastoid

Movers & Antagonists – Exercise 1

1. Serratus posterior superior/Serratus posterior inferior
2. Left rotatores/Right rotatores
3. Right iliocostalis/Left longissimus

Movers & Antagonists – Exercise 2

1. Flexors: relaxed; Extensors: contracting; Type of contraction: eccentric
2. Extensors: relaxed; Flexors: contracting; Type of contraction: eccentric
3. Right lateral flexors: relaxed; Left lateral flexors: contracting; Type of contraction: concentric

Muscle Stabilizations

1. d. Quadratus lumborum
2. a. Erector spinae
3. c. Erector spinae/Transversospinalis
4. b. Serratus posterior superior

You've Got Nerve!

1. Spinal nerves
2. Spinal nerves
3. Spinal nerves
4. Spinal nerves
5. Intercostal nerves
6. Subcostal nerve and intercostal nerves
7. Lumbar plexus

Are You Feeling It? – Palpation

1. Quadratus lumborum
2. Extension and contralateral rotation
3. Erector spinae
4. Between the spinous processes

Clinically Speaking

1. Increased (hyper) lordosis
2. Multifidus (transversus abdominis)
3. Elevation (and anterior tilt)
4. Erector spinae

Muscle Mash-Up

1. Iliocostalis, longissimus, spinalis
2. Semispinalis, multifidus, rotatores
3. Serratus posterior inferior
4. Latissimus dorsi
5. Cervical and lumbar
6. Mastoid process of temporal bone
7. Serratus posterior superior
8. Quadratus lumborum
9. Rotatores
10. Iliocostalis

Mini Case Studies

1. Erector spinae
2. Quadratus lumborum
3. Erector spinae

Crossword Puzzle

Across

5 Semispinalis
11 Intertransversarii
12 Serratus

Down

1 Paraspinal
2 Multifidus
3 Thoracolumbar
4 SP
6 Sacroiliac
7 Quadratus
8 Rotatores
9 Inferior
10 Twelve

Section 2

Know Your Muscles

a. Subcostales
b. External intercostals
c. External abdominal oblique
d. Transversus abdominis
e. Internal intercostals
f. Diaphragm
g. Internal abdominal oblique

h. Levatores costarum
i. Rectus abdominis

What's in a Name?

1. f. External abdominal oblique
2. g. External intercostals
3. h. Diaphragm
4. i. Subcostales
5. j. Internal intercostals
6. d. Internal abdominal oblique
7. e. Levatores costarum
8. b. Transversus abdominis
9. c. Transversus thoracis
10. a. Rectus abdominis

Matching Attachments

1. External intercostals (internal intercostals)
2. Internal intercostals (external intercostals)
3. Levatores costarum
4. Subcostales
5. Transversus thoracis
6. Diaphragm
7. Rectus abdominis
8. Posterior tilt abdominal obliques
9. Internal abdominal obliques
10. Transversus abdominis

The Big Picture – Functional Groups

1. Flexion, trunk, spinal
2. Extension, trunk, spinal
3. Lateral flexion, trunk, spinal
4. Posterior tilt, pelvis, lumbosacral
5. Elevation, ribs, sternocostal and costospinal
6. Depression, ribs, sternocostal and costospinal
7. Posterior tilt of the pelvis at the lumbosacral joint (relative to the spine)

Matching Actions

1. a, h
2. b, g
3. a
4. b
5. b
6. c (a, d)
7. e, i, f (d)
8. e, i, f, h (d)
9. e, i, f, g (d)
10. d

The Long and the Short of It – Exercise 1

1. Shortens
2. Shortens
3. Lengthens
4. Lengthens
5. Shortens

The Long and the Short of It – Exercise 2

1. Shortens: external intercostals, levatores costarum, serratus posterior superior; Lengthens: internal intercostals, subcostales, transversus thoracis, serratus posterior inferior, quadratus lumborum

2. Shortens: internal intercostals, subcostales, transversus thoracis, serratus posterior inferior, quadratus lumborum; Lengthens: external intercostals, levatores costarum, serratus posterior superior
3. Shortens: external abdominal obliques, external intercostals transversospinalis; Lengthens: internal abdominal obliques, internal intercostals
4. Shortens: internal abdominal obliques, internal intercostals; Lengthens: external abdominal obliques, external intercostals, transversospinalis
5. Shortens: rectus abdominis, internal abdominal obliques, external abdominal obliques; Lengthens: erector spinae, transversospinalis, interspinales, quadratus lumborum

Movers & Antagonists – Exercise 1

1. Rectus abdominis/Erector spinae group
2. Left internal intercostals/Right internal intercostals
3. Levatores costarum/Subcostales
4. Left external abdominal oblique/Right internal abdominal oblique

Movers & Antagonists – Exercise 2

1. Right lateral flexors: relaxed; Left lateral flexors: contracting; Type of contraction: eccentric
2. Right rotators: contracting; Left rotators: relaxed; Type of contraction: concentric
3. Left rotators: contracting; Right rotators: relaxed; Type of contraction: concentric

Muscle Stabilizations

1. b. Transversus abdominis
2. d. All of the above
3. c. Diaphragm
4. d. Transversus thoracis

You've Got Nerve!

1. Intercostal nerves
2. Intercostal nerves
3. Spinal nerves
4. Intercostal nerves
5. Intercostal nerves
6. Phrenic nerve
7. Intercostal nerves
8. Intercostal nerves
9. Intercostal nerves
10. Intercostal nerves

Are You Feeling It? – Palpation

1. External abdominal oblique
2. Diaphragm
3. Lateral trunk
4. Rectus abdominis

Clinically Speaking

1. Tendinous inscriptions
2. Intercostals (external and internal)
3. Diaphragm
4. Central tendon (dome)

Muscle Mash-Up

1. Transversus abdominis
2. Central tendon (dome)
3. External abdominal obliques, internal abdominal obliques
4. Levatores costarum
5. External intercostals
6. Rectus abdominis, external abdominal oblique, internal abdominal oblique, transversus abdominis
7. Rectus abdominis
8. Posterior tilt
9. Out
10. Lateral to medial/medial to lateral (horizontally)

Mini Case Studies

1. Transversus abdominis
2. Anterior abdominal wall muscles
3. Intercostals (external and internal)
4. Diaphragm

Crossword Puzzle

Across	Down
1 Aorta	2 Oblique
5 Lifter	3 Subcostales
6 Respiration	4 Splenius
9 Costal	6 Rectus
10 Diaphragm	7 Sheath
11 Corset	8 Intercostals

Section 3

Know Your Muscles

a. Sternocleidomastoid
b. Rectus capitis posterior major
c. Obliquus capitis inferior
d. Splenius capitis
e. Rectus capitis posterior minor
f. Obliquus capitis superior
g. Splenius cervicis

What's in a Name?

1. d. Sternocleidomastoid
2. a. Rectus capitis posterior major
3. e. Rectus capitis posterior minor
4. f. Splenius capitis
5. g. Obliquus capitis inferior
6. c. Splenius cervicis
7. b. Obliquus capitis superior

Matching Attachments

1. Splenius capitis
2. Splenius cervicis
3. Rectus capitis posterior major
4. Rectus capitis posterior minor
5. Obliquus capitis inferior
6. Obliquus capitis superior
7. Sternocleidomastoid

The Big Picture – Functional Groups

1. Flexion, neck, spinal
2. Extension, neck, spinal
3. Right lateral flexion, neck, spinal
4. Flexion of the lower spine relative to the upper spine
5. Extension of the lower spine relative to the upper spine

Matching Actions

1. e, i, k
2. d, h, j
3. a
4. b
5. c
6. b
7. g, f, i, l

The Long and the Short of It – Exercise 1

1. Lengthens
2. Shortens
3. Lengthens
4. Shortens
5. Lengthens

The Long and the Short of It – Exercise 2

1. Shortens: erector spinae, transversospinalis, interspinales, splenius cervicis, splenius capitis, sterno-cleidomastoid, trapezius, levator scapulae; Lengthens: anterior scalene, middle scalene, all hyoids (except stylo-hyoid) longus colli, longus capitis, sternocleidomastoid
2. Shortens: splenius capitis, obliquus capitis inferior, levator scapulae, splenius cervicis; Lengthens: trans-versospinalis, sternocleidomastoid, upper trapezius
3. Shortens: transversospinalis, sternocleidomastoid, upper trapezius; Lengthens: splenius cervicis, splenius capitis, obliquus capitis inferior, levator scapulae
4. Shortens: rectus capitis posterior minor, obliquus capitis superior
5. Shortens: anterior scalene, middle scalene, all hyoids (except stylohyoid), longus colli, longus capitis, ster-nocleidomastoid; Lengthens: erector spinae, trans-versospinalis, interspinalis, splenius cervicis, splenius capitis, sternocleidomastoid, trapezius, levator scapulae

Movers & Antagonists – Exercise 1

1. Left sternocleidomastoid/Left splenius cervicis
2. Right sternocleidomastoid/Right splenius capitis
3. Right semispinalis capitis/Left upper trapezius

Movers & Antagonists – Exercise 2

1. Flexors: relaxed; Extensors: contracting; Type of contraction: eccentric
2. Left lateral flexors: contracting; Right lateral flexors: relaxed; Type of contraction: concentric
3. Left rotators: contracting; Right rotators: relaxed; Type of contraction: concentric

Muscle Stabilizations

1. b. Splenius capitis
2. c. Splenius cervicis
3. a. Rectus capitis posterior major
4. d. Obliquus capitis inferior

You've Got Nerve!

1. Cervical spinal nerves
2. Cervical spinal nerves
3. Suboccipital nerve
4. Suboccipital nerve
5. Suboccipital nerve
6. Suboccipital nerve
7. Spinal accessory nerve (CN XI)

Are You Feeling It? – Palpation

1. Sternocleidomastoid
2. Posterior triangle of the neck
3. Sternal
4. Sternocleidomastoid

Clinically Speaking

1. Suboccipitals
2. Carotid sinus of the common carotid artery
3. Rectus capitis posterior minor
4. Sternocleidomastoid

Muscle Mash-Up

1. Rectus capitis posterior major and minor, obliquus capitis superior and inferior
2. Splenius capitis and cervicis
3. Splenius cervicis
4. Sternocleidomastoid
5. Obliquus capitis inferior
6. Sternal and clavicular
7. Rectus capitis posterior major
8. Head
9. Spinal accessory nerve (CN XI)
10. Splenius capitis

Mini Case Studies

1. Tension headache
2. Suboccipitals (rectus capitis posterior minor, obliquus capitis superior)
3. Cervical flexors
4. You have pressed on the carotid sinus and triggered a reflex to lower blood pressure

Crossword Puzzle

Across	Down
3 Sinus	1 SCM
4 Minor	2 Blood Pressure
5 Whiplash	3 Splenius
7 Sternocleidomastoid	6 Triangle
9 Transverse	8 Major
11 Golf Tee	10 AAJ

Section 4

Know Your Muscles

a. Middle scalene
b. Mylohyoid
c. Posterior scalene
d. Sternohyoid
e. Longus capitis
f. Longus colli
g. Digastric

h. Omohyoid

i. Anterior scalene

What's in a Name?

1. d. Rectus capitis anterior
2. k. Longus capitis
3. i. Mylohyoid
4. c. Geniohyoid
5. m. Stylohyoid
6. h. Longus colli
7. f. Omohyoid
8. e. Posterior scalene
9. g. Anterior scalene
10. b. Thyrohyoid
11. j. Rectus capitis lateralis
12. n. Sternothyroid
13. a. Sternohyoid
14. l. Middle scalene
15. o. Digastric

Matching Attachments

1. Anterior scalene (middle scalene)
2. Middle scalene (anterior scalene)
3. Posterior scalene
4. Digastric
5. Stylohyoid
6. Geniohyoid (mylohyoid)
7. Mylohyoid (geniohyoid)
8. Sternohyoid
9. Sternothyroid
10. Thyrohyoid
11. Omohyoid
12. Longus colli
13. Longus capitis
14. Rectus capitis anterior (rectus capitis lateralis)
15. Rectus capitis lateralis (rectus capitis anterior)

The Big Picture – Functional Groups

1. Flexion, neck, spinal
2. Extension, neck, spinal
3. Left lateral flexion, neck, spinal
4. Elevation, ribs, sternocostal and costospinal
5. Depression, ribs, sternocostal and costospinal
6. Depression, mandible, temporomandibular (TM)
7. Elevation, mandible, temporomandibular (TM)

Matching Actions

1. c, e, i
2. c, e, i
3. e, j
4. g, f, d
5. g
6. g, f, d
7. g, f, d
8. h, c
9. c
10. d
11. a
12. b

The Long and the Short of It – Exercise 1

1. Shortens
2. Lengthens
3. Lengthens
4. Lengthens
5. Shortens

The Long and the Short of It – Exercise 2

1. Shortens: anterior scalene, middle scalene, longus colli, sternocleidomastoid; Lengthens: erector spinae, transversospinalis, interspinales, splenius cervicis, splenius capitis, sternocleidomastoid, trapezius, levator scapulae
2. Shortens: sternohyoid, sternothyroid, thryohyoid, omohyoid; Lengthens: digastric, stylohyoid, geniohyoid, mylohyoid
3. Shortens: anterior scalene, middle scalene; Lengthens: internal intercostals
4. Shortens: erector spinae, transversospinalis, interspinales, splenius cervicis, splenius capitis, sternocleidomastoid, trapezius, levator scapulae; Lengthens: anterior scalene, middle scalene, all hyoids (except stylohyoid), longus colli, sternocleidomastoid
5. Shortens: digastric, stylohyoid, geniohyoid, mylohyoid; Lengthens: sternohyoid, sternothyroid, thyrohyoid, omohyoid

Movers & Antagonists – Exercise 1

1. Right posterior scalene/Left posterior scalene
2. Digastrics/Omohyoid
3. Anterior scalene/Splenius capitis
4. Sternohyoid/Stylohyoid

Movers & Antagonists – Exercise 2

1. Left lateral flexors: relaxed; Right lateral flexors: contracting; Type of contraction: eccentric
2. Flexors: contracting; Extensors: relaxed; Type of contraction: concentric
3. Extensors: contracting; Flexors: relaxed; Type of contraction: concentric

Muscle Stabilizations

1. d. Rectus capitis anterior
2. c. Anterior scalene
3. a. Geniohyoid
4. c. Thyrohyoid
5. b. Posterior scalene

You've Got Nerve!

1. Cervical spinal nerves
2. Cervical spinal nerves
3. Cervical spinal nerves
4. Trigeminal nerve (CN V) and facial nerve (CN VII)
5. Facial nerve (CN VII)
6. Hypoglossal nerve (CN XII)
7. Trigeminal nerve (CN V)
8. Cervical plexus
9. Cervical plexus
10. Hypoglossal nerve (CN XII)
11. Cervical plexus

12. Cervical spinal nerves
13. Cervical spinal nerves
14. Cervical spinal nerves
15. Cervical spinal nerves

Are You Feeling It? – Palpation

1. Scalene group
2. Suprahyoid group
3. Longus
4. Short, quick breaths in through the nose

Clinically Speaking

1. Anterior and middle scalenes
2. Suprahyoids
3. Digastric
4. Subclavian artery

Muscle Mash-Up

1. Transverse processes of the cervical spine
2. Posterior triangle of the neck
3. 1st and 2nd
4. Anterior scalene syndrome, form of thoracic outlet syndrome
5. Blood pressure lowers
6. Anterior, middle, posterior
7. Digastric, stylohyoid, mylohyoid, geniohyoid
8. Sternohyoid, sternothyroid, thyrohyoid, omohyoid
9. Omohyoid
10. Longus capitis

Crossword Puzzle

Across

1 Middle
4 Colli
6 Prevertebral
7 Omohyoid
8 Anterior
11 Whiplash

Down

2 Infrahyoids
3 Digastric
5 Geniohyoid
8 Atlas
9 Thoracic
10 Belly

Mini Case Studies

1. Anterior and middle scalenes
2. Longus colli and capitis
3. Anterior
4. Intrahyoid

Chapters 6–8 Summary Review - Multiple Choice

1. c. Both a and b
2. c. Rotator cuff (SITS)
3. d. Cubital tunnel syndrome
4. d. All of the above
5. b. Scalenes

CHAPTER 9   MUSCLES OF THE HEAD
Coloring & Labeling

Answers for Page Number 174
a. 19
b. 9
c. 15
d. 14
e. 12

f. 17
g. 2
h. 22
i. 18
j. 20
k. 21
l. 8
m. 4
n. 7
o. 3
p. 10
q. 5
r. 1
s. 11
t. 16
u. 23
v. 13
w. 6

Answers for Page Number 175
a. 11
b. 21
c. 25
d. 22
e. 31
f. 23
g. 6
h. 13
i. 17
j. 33
k. 16
l. 3
m. 27
n. 30
o. 26
p. 5
q. 20
r. 28
s. 29
t. 10
u. 1
v. 18
w. 32
x. 4
y. 12
z. 14
aa. 2
bb. 15
cc. 24
dd. 9
ee. 19
ff. 7
gg. 8

Answers for Page Number 176
a. 3
b. 6
c. 5
d. 4
e. 1
f. 2

Section 1

Know Your Muscles

a. Masseter
b. Medial pterygoid
c. Auricularis group
d. Lateral pterygoid
e. Temporalis
f. Temporoparietalis
g. Occipitofrontalis

What's in a Name?

1. h. Occipitofrontalis
2. b. Masseter
3. g. Auricularis posterior
4. a. Temporalis
5. c. Lateral pterygoid
6. d. Medial pterygoid
7. i. Temporoparietalis
8. e. Auricularis anterior
9. f. Auricularis superior

Matching Attachments

1. Temporalis
2. Masseter
3. Lateral pterygoid
4. Medial pterygoid
5. Auricularis anterior
6. Auricularis superior
7. Auricularis posterior
8. Occipitofrontalis
9. Temporoparietalis

The Big Picture – Functional Groups

1. Depression, mandible, temporomandibular (TM)
2. Elevation, mandible, temporomandibular (TM)
3. Contralateral deviation, mandible, temporomandibular (TM)
4. Protraction, mandible, temporomandibular (TM)
5. Retraction, mandible, temporomandibular (TM)

Matching Actions

1. a
2. a
3. b, c
4. a, b, c
5. e
6. f
7. g
8. d
9. f

The Long and the Short of It – Exercise 1

1. Shortens
2. Lengthens
3. Lengthens
4. Shortens
5. Shortens

The Long and the Short of It – Exercise 2

1. Shortens: temporalis, masseter, medial pterygoid; Lengthens: digastric, mylohyoid, geniohyoid
2. Shortens: digastric, mylohyoid, geniohyoid; Lengthens: temporalis, masseter, medial pterygoid
3. Shortens: auricularis anterior; Lengthens: auricularis posterior
4. Shortens: auricularis posterior; Lengthens: auricularis anterior
5. Shortens: lateral pterygoid, medial pterygoid;

Movers & Antagonists – Exercise 1

1. Temporalis/Digastric
2. Right lateral pterygoid/Left medial pterygoid

Movers & Antagonists – Exercise 2

1. Elevators: contracting; Depressors: relaxed; Type of contraction: concentric
2. Protractors: contracting; Retractors: relaxed; Type of contraction: concentric
3. Right lateral deviators: contracting; Left lateral deviators: relaxed; Type of contraction: concentric

Muscle Stabilizations

1. d. Medial pterygoid
2. b. Masseter

You've Got Nerve!

1. Trigeminal nerve (CN V)
2. Trigeminal nerve (CN V)
3. Trigeminal nerve (CN V)
4. Trigeminal nerve (CN V)
5. Facial nerve (CN VII)
6. Facial nerve (CN VII)
7. Facial nerve (CN VII)
8. Facial nerve (CN VII)
9. Facial nerve (CN VII)

Are You Feeling It? – Palpation

1. Temporalis
2. Lateral pterygoid
3. Alternately clench the teeth and relax the jaw
4. Elevate the eyebrows

Clinically Speaking

1. They are parallel/identical
2. Temporalis
3. Lateral pterygoid
4. Masseter
5. Auricularis group

Muscle Mash-Up

1. Occipitofrontalis
2. Temporalis, masseter, lateral pterygoid, medial pterygoid
3. Medial pterygoid
4. Lateral pterygoid, medial pterygoid
5. Occipitalis, frontalis
6. Between the zygomatic arch and the angle of the mandible
7. Protraction and contralateral deviation of the mandible
8. Medial pterygoid
9. Auricularis anterior, posterior, and superior
10. Galea aponeurotica

301

Mini Case Studies

1. Lateral pterygoid
2. Temporalis, masseter, lateral pterygoid, medial pterygoid
3. Occipitofrontalis
4. Masseter

Crossword Puzzle

Across

1 Fossa
4 Masseter
10 Auricularis
11 CNV
12 Pterygoid

Down

2 Sphenoid
3 TMJ
5 Superior
6 Elevate
7 Mastication
8 Facial
9 Elevation

Sections 2

Know Your Muscles

a. Orbicularis oculi
b. Procerus
c. Levator anguli oris
d. Platysma
e. Corrugator supercilii
f. Zygomaticus major
g. Levator labii superioris
h. Buccinator

What's in a Name?

1. j. Depressor anguli oris
2. d. Levator anguli oris
3. f. Buccinator
4. e. Levator labii superioris
5. k. Orbicularis oculi
6. a. Levator palpebrae superioris
7. q. Zygomaticus minor
8. i. Mentalis
9. h. Depressor septi nasi
10. o. Nasalis
11. n. Corrugator supercilii
12. p. Levator labii superioris alaeque nasi
13. b. Zygomaticus major
14. r. Platysma
15. g. Depressor labii inferioris
16. c. Procerus
17. m. Orbicularis oris
18. l. Risorius

Matching Attachments

1. Orbicularis oculi
2. Levator palpebrae superioris
3. Corrugator supercilii
4. Procerus
5. Nasalis
6. Depressor septi nasi
7. Levator labii superioris alaeque nasi
8. Levator labii superioris
9. Zygomaticus minor

10. Zygomaticus major
11. Levator anguli oris
12. Risorius
13. Buccinator
14. Depressor anguli oris
15. Depressor labii inferioris
16. Mentalis
17. Orbicularis oris
18. Platysma

The Big Picture – Functional Groups

1. Elevation (up)
2. Depression (down)
3. Laterally (to the side)
4. Elevation (up)
5. Depression (down)

Matching Actions

1. a
2. b
3. c
4. d, e
5. f, g
6. f
7. g, h
8. h
9. h
10. n
11. n
12. p
13. q
14. o
15. j
16. i, k, l
17. r, m
18. s

The Long and the Short of It – Exercise 1

1. Lengthens
2. Shortens
3. Lengthens
4. Shortens
5. Lengthens

The Long and the Short of It – Exercise 2

1. Shortens: nasalis, depressor septi nasi; Lengthens: nasalis, levator labii superioris alaeque nasi
2. Shortens: zygomaticus major, levator anguli oris; Lengthens: depressor anguli oris
3. Shortens: mentalis; Lengthens: depressor labii inferioris
4. Shortens: depressor anguli oris; Lengthens: zygomaticus major, levator anguli oris
5. Shortens: nasalis, levator labii superioris alaeque nasi; Lengthens: nasalis, depressor septi nasi

Movers & Antagonists – Exercise 1

1. Occipitofrontalis/Procerus
2. Auricularis anterior/Auricularis posterior
3. Nasalis/Depressor septi nasi
4. Levator anguli oris/Depressor anguli oris

302

You've Got Nerve!

1. Facial nerve (CN VII)
2. Facial nerve (CN VII)
3. Facial nerve (CN VII)
4. Facial nerve (CN VII)
5. Facial nerve (CN VII)
6. Facial nerve (CN VII)
7. Facial nerve (CN VII)
8. Facial nerve (CN VII)
9. Facial nerve (CN VII)
10. Facial nerve (CN VII)
11. Facial nerve (CN VII)
12. Facial nerve (CN VII)
13. Facial nerve (CN VII)
14. Facial nerve (CN VII)
15. Facial nerve (CN VII)
16. Facial nerve (CN VII)
17. Facial nerve (CN VII)
18. Facial nerve (CN VII)

Are You Feeling It? – Palpation

1. Somewhat forcefully close the eye
2. Corrugator supercilii
3. Procerus
4. Buccinator
5. Forcefully depress and draw the lower lip laterally

Clinically Speaking

1. Orbicularis oculi
2. It paralyzes the musculature
3. Levator anguli oris
4. Platysma
5. Buccinators
6. Mentalis

Muscle Mash-Up

1. Procerus
2. Zygomaticus minor and major
3. Levator labii superioris alaequae nasi
4. Orbicularis oculi, levator palpebrae superioris, corrugator supercilii
5. Procerus, nasalis, depressor septi nasi (levator labii superioris alaeque nasi)
6. Levator labii superioris alaeque nasi
7. Buccinator
8. Facial (CN VII)
9. Orbicularis oculi
10. Bright sunlight

Crossword Puzzle

Across	Down
2 Constricts	1 Orbicularis
3 Maxilla	4 Major
5 Caninus	6 Nasalis
8 Nasi	7 Pout
9 Risorius	10 Major
11 Labii	
12 Sorrow	

Mini Case Studies

1. Orbicularis oculi
2. Buccinator
3. Orbicular oris
4. He is very expressive with facial musculature

CHAPTER 10   MUSCLES OF THE PELVIS AND THIGH

Coloring & Labeling

Answers for Page Number 198

a. 25
b. 4
c. 8
d. 1
e. 21
f. 11
g. 30
h. 16
i. 15
j. 22
k. 23
l. 6
m. 24
n. 5
o. 18
p. 32
q. 27
r. 7
s. 33
t. 12
u. 26
v. 9
w. 28
x. 2
y. 29
z. 31
aa. 20
bb. 10
cc. 17
dd. 13
ee. 14
ff. 19
gg. 3

Answers for Page Number 199

a. 25
b. 13
c. 6
d. 3
e. 22
f. 29
g. 15
h. 14
i. 27
j. 11
k. 7
l. 12
m. 1
n. 28
o. 17

p. 23
q. 30
r. 26
s. 24
t. 18
u. 19
v. 4
w. 10
x. 21
y. 8
z. 9
aa. 31
bb. 5
cc. 2
dd. 16
ee. 20

Answers for Page Number 200
a. 20
b. 23
c. 12
d. 18
e. 14
f. 24
g. 5
h. 1
i. 17
j. 19
k. 4
l. 7
m. 26
n. 13
o. 8
p. 2
q. 9
r. 11
s. 16
t. 10
u. 22
v. 6
w. 3
x. 15
y. 21
z. 25

Answers for Page Number 201
a. 8
b. 4
c. 15
d. 2
e. 4
f. 7
g. 14
h. 1
i. 13
j. 10
k. 9
l. 2
m. 3
n. 11
o. 5

Section 3

Know Your Muscles
a. Gluteus minimus
b. Piriformis
c. Inferior gemellus
d. Obturator internus
e. Gluteus maximus
f. Obturator externus
g. Gluteus medius
h. Superior gemellus
i. Quadratus femoris

What's in a Name?
1. h. Obturator internus
2. f. Obturator externus
3. e. Gluteus minimus
4. g. Gluteus medius
5. d. Inferior gemellus
6. e. Superior gemellus
7. b. Quadratus femoris
8. a. Gluteus maximus
9. i. Piriformis

Matching Attachments
1. Gluteus maximus
2. Gluteus medius (gluteus minimus)
3. Gluteus minimus (gluteus medius)
4. Piriformis
5. Superior gemellus
6. Obturator internus
7. Inferior gemellus
8. Obturator externus
9. Quadratus femoris

The Big Picture – Functional Groups
1. Flexion, thigh, hip; anterior tilt, pelvis, hip
2. Extension, thigh, hip; posterior tilt, pelvis, hip
3. Abduction, thigh, hip
4. Adduction, thigh, hip
5. Posterior tilt, pelvis, hip
6. Contralateral rotation, pelvis, hip

Matching Actions
1. b, d, f, g, i, j
2. a, b, d, e, f, h, i, j, k
3. a, b, d, e, f, h, i, j, k
4. c, d, e, j
5. d, j
6. d, j
7. d, j
8. d, j
9. d, j

The Long and the Short of It – Exercise 1
1. Lengthens
2. Shortens
3. Lengthens
4. Shortens
5. Shortens

The Long and the Short of It – Exercise 2

1. Shortens: gluteus medius, gluteus minimus, tensor fasciae latae, sartorius, iliacus, psoas major, pectineus, gracilis, adductor longus, adductor brevis, rectus femoris; Lengthens: gluteus medius, gluteus minimus, gluteus maximus, adductor magnus, biceps femoris, semitendinosus, semimembranosus
2. Shortens: gluteus medius, gluteus minimus, gluteus maximus, adductor magnus, biceps femoris, semitendinosus, semimembranosus; Lengthens: gluteus medius, gluteus minimus, tensor fasciae latae, sartorius, iliacus, psoas major, pectineus, gracilis, adductor longus, adductor brevis, rectus femoris
3. Shortens: gluteus medius, gluteus minimus, piriformis, tensor fasciae latae; Lengthens: gluteus maximus, gluteus medius, gluteus minimus, piriformis, superior gemellus, obturator internus, inferior gemellus, obturator externus, quadratus femoris, sartorius, iliacus, psoas major
4. Shortens: gluteus maximus, pectineus, gracilis, adductor longus, adductor brevis, adductor magnus; Lengthens: gluteus maximus, gluteus medius, gluteus minimus, tensor fasciae latae, sartorius
5. Shortens: gluteus maximus, gluteus medius, gluteus minimus, piriformis, superior gemellus, obturator internus, inferior gemellus, obturator externus, quadratus femoris, sartorius, iliacus, psoas major; Lengthens: gluteus medius, gluteus minimus, piriformis, tensor fasciae latae

Movers & Antagonists – Exercise 1

1. Anterior gluteus medius/Posterior gluteus medius
2. Piriformis /Anterior gluteus minimus
3. Gluteus maximus/Anterior gluteus medius
4. Upper gluteus maximus/Lower gluteus maximus

Movers & Antagonists – Exercise 2

1. Flexors: contracting; Extensors: relaxed; Type of contraction: concentric
2. Extensors: contracting; Flexors: relaxed; Type of contraction: concentric
3. Lateral rotators: contracting; Medial rotators: relaxed; Type of contraction: concentric

Muscle Stabilizations

1. d. All of the above
2. b. Piriformis
3. d. Piriformis

You've Got Nerve!

1. Inferior gluteal nerve
2. Superior gluteal nerve
3. Superior gluteal nerve
4. Nerve to piriformis (of the Lumbosacral plexus)
5. Nerve to obturator internus (of the Lumbosacral plexus)
6. Nerve to obturator internus (of the Lumbosacral plexus)
7. Nerve to quadratus femoris (of the Lumbosacral plexus)
8. The obturator nerve
9. Nerve to quadratus femoris (of the Lumbosacral plexus)

Are You Feeling It? – Palpation

1. Laterally rotate and extend the thigh
2. Side-lying
3. Between the greater trochanter of the femur and the sacrum, immediately lateral to the sacrum, halfway between the PSIS and apex of the sacrum
4. Lateral to the lateral border of the ischial tuberosity
5. Distal thigh

Clinically Speaking

1. Medius
2. Gluteus medius
3. Gluteus medius and minimus on that side
4. Medial rotation of the thigh
5. Part or all of it pierces the piriformis muscle
6. Piriformis syndrome

Muscle Mash-Up

1. Gluteus maximus
2. Gluteus maximus, medius, and minimus
3. Piriformis, superior and inferior gemellus, obturator internus and externus, quadratus femoris
4. Flexion of the thigh and anterior tilt of the pelvis at the hip joint
5. Gluteus minimus
6. Lateral pelvis
7. Contralateral rotation of the pelvis at the hip joint
8. Piriformis
9. Quadratus femoris
10. Gluteus maximus

Crossword Puzzle

Across

4 Pelvis
7 Medius
9 Maximus
10 Obturator
12 Superior

Down

1 Gemellus
2 Deep
3 Minimus
5 Piriformis
6 Quadratus
8 ITB
11 TFL

Mini Case Studies

1. Right gluteus medius
2. With the client's thigh first flexed, then either horizontally flex (horizontally adduct) or laterally rotate it
3. Lateral rotators of the thigh at the hip joint
4. Sacroiliac joint on the side of the spasm

Section 2

Know Your Muscles

a. Psoas major
b. Iliacus
c. Tensor fasciae latae
d. Gracilis
e. Adductor magnus
f. Psoas minor
g. Pectineus
h. Adductor longus
i. Sartorius

What's in a Name?

1. g. Pectineus
2. j. Psoas minor
3. c. Adductor brevis
4. h. Psoas major
5. e. Iliacus
6. a. Sartorius
7. f. Adductor magnus
8. b. Adductor longus
9. d. Gracilis
10. i. Tensor fasciae latae

Matching Attachments

1. Tensor fasciae latae
2. Sartorius
3. Iliacus
4. Psoas major
5. Psoas minor
6. Pectineus
7. Gracilis
8. Adductor longus (adductor brevis)
9. Adductor brevis (adductor longus)
10. Adductor magnus

The Big Picture – Functional Groups

1. Flexion, thigh, hip joint; anterior tilt, pelvis, hip joint
2. Extension, thigh, hip joint; posterior tilt, pelvis, hip joint
3. Abduction, thigh, hip joint; depression (lateral tilt), same-side pelvis, hip joint
4. Adduction, thigh, hip joint; elevation, same-side pelvis, hip joint
5. Flexion, trunk, spinal joints
6. Anterior tilt, pelvis, hip joint

Matching Actions

1. a, d, f, h, j
2. a, d, g, h, b
3. a, g, h
4. a, g, h, c
5. c, i
6. e, a, h
7. e, a, h, b
8. e, a, h
9. e, a, h
10. e, i, k

The Long and the Short of It – Exercise 1

1. Lengthens
2. Shortens
3. Shortens
4. Shortens
5. Lengthens

The Long and the Short of It – Exercise 2

1. Shortens: gluteus medius, gluteus minimus, gluteus maximus, adductor magnus, biceps femoris, semitendinosus, semimembranosus; Lengthens: gluteus medius, gluteus minimus, tensor fasciae latae, sartorius, iliacus, psoas major, pectineus, gracilis, adductor longus, adductor brevis, rectus femoris
2. Shortens: gluteus medius, gluteus minimus, tensor fasciae latae, sartorius, iliacus, psoas major, pectineus, gracilis, adductor longus, adductor brevis, rectus femoris; Lengthens: gluteus medius, gluteus minimus, gluteus maximus, psoas minor, adductor magnus, biceps femoris, semitendinosus, semimembranosus
3. Shortens: gluteus medius, gluteus minimus, piriformis, tensor fasciae latae; Lengthens: gluteus maximus, gluteus medius, gluteus minimus, piriformis, superior gemellus, obturator internus, inferior gemellus, obturator externus, quadratus femoris, sartorius, iliacus, psoas major
4. Shortens: gluteus medius, gluteus minimus, tensor fasciae latae, sartorius, iliacus, psoas major, pectineus, gracilis, adductor longus, adductor brevis, rectus femoris; Lengthens: gluteus medius, gluteus minimus, gluteus maximus, adductor magnus, biceps femoris, semitendinosus, semimembranosus
5. Shortens: gluteus maximus, gluteus medius, gluteus minimus, tensor fasciae latae, sartorius; Lengthens: gluteus maximus, pectineus, gracilis, adductor longus, adductor brevis, adductor magnus

Movers & Antagonists – Exercise 1

1. Gluteus maximus/Iliopsoas
2. Sartorius/Tensor fasciae latae
3. Adductor magnus/Posterior gluteus medius
4. Sartorius/Gluteus maximus

Movers & Antagonists – Exercise 2

1. Adductors: relaxed; Abductors: contracting; Type of contraction: eccentric
2. Adductors: contracting; Abductors: relaxed; Type of contraction: concentric
3. Flexors: relaxed; Extensors: contracting; Type of contraction: eccentric

Muscle Stabilizations

1. a. Tensor fasciae latae
2. a. Gracilis
3. c. Psoas minor
4. b. Adductor longus

You've Got Nerve!

1. Superior gluteal nerve
2. Femoral nerve
3. Femoral nerve
4. Lumbar plexus
5. L1 spinal nerve
6. Femoral nerve
7. Obturator nerve
8. Obturator nerve
9. Obturator nerve
10. Obturator nerve and sciatic nerve

Are You Feeling It? – Palpation

1. Medial rotation and flexion of the thigh at the hip joint
2. Lateral rotation and flexion of the thigh at the hip joint
3. Distal thigh
4. Halfway between the ASIS and umbilicus, lateral to the rectus abdominis
5. Adductor longus
6. Gracilis and medial hamstrings (semitendinosus and semimembranosus)

Clinically Speaking

1. Iliotibial band friction syndrome
2. Sartorius, gracilis, semitendinosus
3. Femoral nerve, artery, and vein
4. Aorta
5. Sartorius and adductor longus
6. Adductor magnus

Muscle Mash-Up

1. Psoas major, iliacus
2. Adductor longus, brevis and magnus, pectineus, gracilis
3. Gracilis
4. Adductor magnus
5. Tensor fasciae latae, gluteus maximus
6. Pubic bone
7. Psoas major
8. Adductor longus
9. Pectineus
10. Extension of the thigh and posterior tilt of the pelvis at the hip joint
11. Anterior and posterior
12. Roots of the lumbar plexus

Mini Case Studies

1. Meralgia paresthetica, sartorius
2. Increased anterior tilt of the pelvis/hyperlordosis/swayback
3. Adductor
4. Psoas minor syndrome

Crossword Puzzle

Across	Down
1 TFL	2 Lesser
3 Swayback	4 Psoas Minor
7 Gracilis	5 Femoral
9 Goose Foot	6 Sartorius
10 Thirty	8 Inguinal
11 Psoas Major	
12 PES	

Section 3

Know Your Muscles

a. Vastus lateralis
b. Articularis genus
c. Vastus medialis
d. Semimembranosus
e. Semitendinosus
f. Vastus intermedius
g. Biceps femoris
h. Rectus femoris

What's in a Name?

1. b. Semimembranosus
2. c. Semitendinosus
3. g. Biceps femoris
4. f. Rectus femoris
5. d. Vastus lateralis
6. h. Vastus intermedius
7. a. Vastus medialis
8. e. Articularis genus

Matching Attachments

1. Rectus femoris
2. Vastus lateralis (vastus medialus)
3. Vastus medialis (vastus lateralis)
4. Vastus intermedius
5. Articularis genus
6. Biceps femoris
7. Semitendinosus
8. Semimembranosus

The Big Picture – Functional Groups

1. Flexion, thigh, hip; anterior tilt, pelvis, hip
2. Extension, thigh, hip; posterior tilt, pelvis, hip
3. Extension, leg, knee
4. Flexion, leg, knee
5. Anterior tilt, pelvis, hip
6. Extension, thigh, knee

Matching Actions

1. a, b, d, f
2. a, b
3. a, b
4. a, b
5. h
6. e, c, g
7. e, c, g
8. e, c, g

The Long and the Short of It – Exercise 1

1. Shortens
2. Shortens
3. Lengthens
4. Shortens
5. Lengthens

The Long and the Short of It – Exercise 2

1. Shortens: rectus femoris, vastus lateralis, vastus medialis, vastus intermedius; Lengthens: biceps femoris, semitendinosus, semimembranosus, sartorius, gracilis
2. Shortens: gluteus medius, gluteus minimus, gluteus maximus, psoas minor, adductor magnus, biceps femoris, semitendinosus, semimembranosus; Lengthens: gluteus medius, gluteus minimus, tensor fasciae latae, sartorius, iliacus, psoas major, pectineus, gracilis, adductor longus, adductor brevis, rectus femoris

3. Shortens: gluteus medius, gluteus minimus, tensor fasciae latae, sartorius, iliacus, psoas major, pectineus, gracilis, adductor longus, adductor brevis, rectus femoris; Lengthens: gluteus medius, gluteus minimus, gluteus maximus, adductor magnus, biceps femoris, semitendinosus, semimembranosus

4. Shortens: biceps femoris, semitendinosus, semimembranosus, sartorius, gracilis; Lengthens: rectus femoris, vastus lateralis, vastus medialis, vastus intermedius

5. Shortens: gluteus medius, gluteus minimus, tensor fasciae latae, sartorius, iliacus, psoas major, pectineus, gracilis, adductor longus, adductor brevis, rectus femoris; Lengthens: gluteus medius, gluteus minimus, gluteus maximus, adductor magnus, biceps femoris, semitendinosus, semimembranosus

Movers & Antagonists – Exercise 1

1. Hamstring group/Quadriceps femoris group
2. Vastus lateralis/Semitendinosus
3. Rectus femoris/Gluteus maximus
4. Biceps femoris/Iliopsoas

Movers & Antagonists – Exercise 2

1. Extensors: relaxed; Flexors: contracting; Type of contraction: eccentric
2. Extensors: contracting; Flexors: relaxed; Type of contraction: concentric
3. Lateral rotators: contracting; Medial rotators: relaxed; Type of contraction: concentric

Muscle Stabilizations

1. c. rectus femoris
2. d. vastus intermedius
3. a. articularis genus

You've Got Nerve!

1. Femoral nerve
2. Femoral nerve
3. Femoral nerve
4. Femoral nerve
5. Femoral nerve
6. Sciatic nerve
7. Sciatic nerve
8. Sciatic nerve

Are You Feeling It? – Palpation

1. Extension of the knee joint
2. Ischial tuberosity
3. Distal leg
4. Vastus lateralis
5. Flexion of the leg at the knee joint (extension of the thigh at the hip joint)
6. Head of fibula

Clinically Speaking

1. Sartorius, gracilis, semitendinosus
2. Semitendinosus
3. Semimembranosus
4. Distal aspect (vastus medialis oblique fibers)
5. Vastus lateralis

Muscle Mash-Up

1. Rectus femoris, vastus lateralis, medialis, and intermedius
2. Biceps femoris, semitendinosus, semimembranosus
3. Semitendinosus, semimembranosus
4. Long and short
5. Articularis genus
6. Ischial tuberosity
7. Rectus femoris
8. Short head of the biceps femoris
9. Vastus lateralis
10. Vastus intermedius
11. Linea aspera of the femur
12. Semimembranosus

Crossword Puzzle

Across

3 VMO
4 Straight
6 Superficial
9 AIIS
11 Extension

Down

1 Posterior
2 Patella
5 Tuberosity
7 Sartorius
8 Knee
10 Semi
12 Sciatic

Mini Case Studies

1. Vastus lateralis, tensor fasciae latae, gluteus maximus
2. Quadriceps femoris
3. Hamstrings
4. Semimembranosus

CHAPTER 11   MUSCLES OF THE LEG AND FOOT

Answers for Page Number 236

a. 13
b. 9
c. 12
d. 10
e. 3
f. 15
g. 7
h. 14
i. 8
j. 11
k. 6
l. 4
m. 5
n. 2
o. 1

Answers for Page Number 237

a. 3
b. 14
c. 13
d. 19
e. 18
f. 9
g. 12
h. 8
i. 2

j. 17
k. 4
l. 5
m. 20
n. 6
o. 15
p. 1
q. 7
r. 10
s. 11
t. 16

Answers for Page Number 238
a. 12
b. 19
c. 16
d. 8
e. 2
f. 23
g. 15
h. 21
i. 13
j. 4
k. 9
l. 22
m. 6
n. 22
o. 14
p. 5
q. 3
r. 10
s. 11
t. 17
u. 1
v. 18
w. 7

Answers for Page Number 239
a. 4
b. 13
c. 18
d. 14
e. 12
f. 8
g. 3
h. 9
i. 5
j. 11
k. 16
l. 15
m. 2
n. 6
o. 17
p. 1
q. 7
r. 10

Answers for Page Number 240
a. 5
b. 1
c. 6
d. 4

e. 2
f. 3

Answers for Page Number 241
a. 17
b. 4
c. 7
d. 14
e. 8
f. 3
g. 9
h. 10
i. 11
j. 1
k. 2
l. 13
m. 6
n. 16
o. 12
p. 5
q. 15

Answers for Page Number 242
a. 11
b. 1
c. 10
d. 6
e. 9
f. 7
g. 4
h. 3
i. 2
j. 6
k. 7
l. 12

Section 1

Know Your Muscles

a. Extensor digitorum longus
b. Fibularis brevis
c. Extensor hallucis longus
d. Fibularis longus
e. Tibialis anterior
f. Fibularis tertius

What's in a Name?

1. f. Extensor digitorum longus
2. b. Fibularis brevis
3. a. Fibularis tertius
4. e. Extensor hallucis longus
5. c. Tibialis anterior
6. d. Fibularis longus

Matching Attachments

1. Tibialis anterior
2. Extensor hallucis longus
3. Extensor digitorum longus
4. Fibularis longus
5. Fibularis brevis
6. Fibularis tertius

309

Answer Key

The Big Picture – Functional Groups

1. Dorsiflexion, foot, ankle joint
2. Plantarflexion, foot, ankle joint
3. Inversion, foot, subtalar joint
4. Eversion, foot, subtalar joint
5. The leg moves toward the foot at the ankle joint instead of the foot moving toward the leg

Matching Actions

1. a, c
2. e, a, c
3. f, d, a
4. b, d
5. b, d
6. a, d

The Long and the Short of It – Exercise 1

1. Lengthens
2. Lengthens
3. Shortens
4. Lengthens
5. Shortens

The Long and the Short of It – Exercise 2

1. Shortens: extensor digitorum longus, fibularis longus, fibularis brevis, fibularis tertius; Lengthens: tibialis anterior, extensor hallucis longus, tibialis posterior, flexor digitorum longus, flexor hallucis longus
2. Shortens: tibialis anterior, extensor hallucis longus, tibialis posterior, flexor digitorum longus, flexor hallucis longus; Lengthens: extensor digitorum longus, extensor hallucis longus, fibularis longus, fibularis brevis, fibularis tertius
3. Shortens: tibialis anterior, extensor digitorum longus, extensor hallucis longus, fibuarlis tertius; Lengthens: fibularis longus, fibularis brevis, gastrocnemius, soleus, plantaris, tibialis posterior, flexor digitorum longus, flexor hallucis longus
4. Shortens: fibularis longus, fibularis brevis, gastrocnemius, soleus, plantaris, tibialis posterior, flexor digitorum longus, flexor hallucis longus; Lengthens: tibialis anterior, extensor digitorum longus, extensor hallucis longus, fibularis tertius
5. Shortens: extensor hallucis longus; Lengthens: flexor hallucis longus

Movers & Antagonists – Exercise 1

1. Tibialis anterior/Fibularis longus
2. Fibularis longus/Tibialis anterior
3. Fibularis brevis/Extensor digitorum longus
4. Extensor hallucis longus/Fibularis tertius

Movers & Antagonists – Exercise 2

1. Dorsiflexors: contracting; Plantarflexors: relaxed; Type of contraction: concentric
2. Plantarflexors: relaxed; Dorsiflexors: contracting; Type of contraction: eccentric
3. Inverters: contracting; Everters: relaxed; Type of contraction: concentric

Muscle Stabilizations

1. d. All of the above
2. b. Extensor hallucis longus
3. d. Extensor digitorum longus
4. d. None of the above

You've Got Nerve!

1. Deep fibular nerve
2. Deep fibular nerve
3. Deep fibular nerve
4. Superficial fibular nerve
5. Superficial fibular nerve
6. Deep fibular nerve

Are You Feeling It? – Palpation

1. Dorsiflexion of the foot at the ankle joint, inversion of the foot at the subtalar joint
2. Dorsal surface of the distal phalanx of the big toe
3. No. The extensor hallucis longus will isometrically contract.
4. Eversion of the foot at the subtalar joint (inversion of the foot at the ankle joint)
5. Look immediately lateral to the tendon of extensor digitorum longus to the little toe for the fibularis tertius tendon

Clinically Speaking

1. Tibialis anterior
2. Tibialis anterior
3. Extensor digitorum longus
4. Fibularis longus

Muscle Mash-Up

1. Fibularis longus, brevis, and tertius
2. Tibialis anterior (extensor hallucis longus)
3. Fibularis longus and brevis
4. Tibialis anterior, extensor digitorum longus, extensor hallucis longus, fibularis tertius
5. Fibularis longus and brevis
6. Extensor hallucis longus
7. Fibularis longus, fibularis brevis
8. Tibialis anterior and fibularis longus
9. Fibularis
10. Extensor digitorum longus

Mini Case Studies

1. Anterior shin splints; tibialis anterior
2. Fibularis group (everters)
3. Inverters of the foot at the subtalar joint
4. Tibialis anterior and fibularis longus (stirrup muscles); also tibialis posterior

Crossword Puzzle

Across	Down
2 Longus	1 Medial foot
5 Brevis	3 Sidelying
7 Hallucis	4 Tibialis anterior
9 Dorsiflexion	6 Deep fibular
10 Gait	8 Tertius
11 Fibularis	
12 Digitorum	

Know Your Muscles

a. Soleus
b. Plantaris
c. Flexor digitorum longus
d. Popliteus
e. Flexor hallucis longus
f. Gastrocnemius
g. Tibialis posterior

What's in a Name?

1. b. Flexor hallucis longus
2. e. Flexor digitorum longus
3. g. Gastrocnemius
4. f. Soleus
5. c. Popliteus
6. a. Tibialis posterior
7. d. Plantaris

Matching Attachments

1. Gastrocnemius
2. Soleus
3. Plantaris
4. Tibialis posterior
5. Flexor digitorum longus
6. Flexor hallucis longus
7. Popliteus

The Big Picture – Functional Groups

1. Plantarflexion, foot, ankle joint
2. Inversion, foot, subtalar joint
3. Flexion, leg, knee joint
4. Flexion, toes
5. Extension, toes
6. Dorsiflexion, leg, ankle

Matching Actions

1. a, b
2. a
3. a, b
4. a, c
5. a, c, d
6. a, c, e
7. b, f, g

The Long and the Short of It – Exercise 1

1. Lengthens
2. Shortens
3. Shortens
4. Lengthens
5. Lengthens

The Long and the Short of It – Exercise 2

1. Shortens: popliteus; Lengthens: biceps femoris
2. Shortens: tibialis anterior, extensor hallucis longus, extensor digitorum longus fibularis tertius; Lengthens: fibularis longus, fibularis brevis, gastrocnemius, soleus, plantaris, tibialis posterior, flexor digitorum longus, flexor hallucis longus
3. Shortens: flexor digitorum longus, flexor digitorum brevis, lumbricals pedis, quadratus plantae; Lengthens: extensor digitorum longus, extensor digitorum brevis, lumbricals pedis
4. Shortens: flexor hallucis longus, flexor hallucis brevis; Lengthens: extensor hallucis longus, extensor hallucis brevis
5. Shortens: tibialis anterior, extensor hallucis longus, tibialis posterior, flexor digitorum longus, flexor hallucis longus; Lengthens: extensor digitorum longus, fibularis longus, fibularis brevis, fibularis tertius

Movers & Antagonists – Exercise 1

1. Gastrocnemius/Tibialis anterior
2. Extensor digitorum longus/Flexor digitorum longus
3. Tibialis posterior/Fibularis longus
4. Extensor hallucis longus/Flexor hallucis longus

Movers & Antagonists – Exercise 2

1. Plantarflexors: relaxed; Dorsiflexors: contracting; Type of contraction: eccentric
2. Medial rotators: contracting; Lateral rotators: relaxed; Type of contraction: concentric
3. Lateral rotators: contracting; Medial rotators: relaxed; Type of contraction: concentric

Muscle Stabilizations

1. d. Flexor digitorum longus
2. b. Gastrocnemius
3. a. Popliteus
4. c. Flexor hallucis longus

You've Got Nerve!

1. Tibial nerve
2. Tibial nerve
3. Tibial nerve
4. Tibial nerve
5. Tibial nerve
6. Tibial nerve
7. Tibial nerve

Are You Feeling It? – Palpation

1. Flexed to approximately 90 degrees
2. Extended
3. Immediately posterior and distal to the medial malleolus of the tibia
4. Distal medial leg between the soleus and tibia
5. Medial rotation of the leg at the knee joint
6. Medial shaft of tibia, at level of tibial tuberosity

Clinically Speaking

1. Posterior ankle/heel
2. Soleus
3. Tibialis posterior
4. Tibialis posterior
5. Popliteus

Muscle Mash-Up

1. Medial and lateral
2. Lateral and medial leg

3. Full extension
4. Calcaneus via the calcaneal (Achilles) tendon
5. Tibialis posterior, flexor digitorum longus, flexor hallucis longus
6. Medial and lateral heads of gastrocnemius, and soleus
7. Their distal tendons all cross posterior and distal to the medial malleolus of the tibia
8. Distal medial leg
9. Tibialis posterior, flexor digitorum longus, flexor hallucis longus, popliteus
10. Gastrocnemius, soleus, plantaris

Crossword Puzzle

Across

1 Popliteus
3 Tibial
7 Harry
8 Gastrocnemius
10 Tom

Down

1 Plantaris
2 Dick
4 Paris
5 Calcaneal
6 Laterally
8 Gastro
9 Invert

Mini Case Studies

1. Plantarflexors, primarily triceps surae (gastrocnemius and soleus)
2. Stretch the client into dorsiflexion at the ankle joint, with the knee joint flexed (for soleus) and extended (for gastrocnemius)
3. Posterior shin splints (involving the tibialis posterior)
4. Popliteus

Section 3

Know Your Muscles

a. Abductor hallucis
b. Extensor hallucis brevis
c. Flexor digitorum brevis
d. Dorsal interossei pedis
e. Adductor hallucis
f. Plantar interossei
g. Abductor digiti minimi pedis
h. Flexor hallucis brevis
i. Quadratus plantae

What's in a Name?

1. k. Plantar interossei
2. e. Flexor digitorum brevis
3. g. Quadratus plantae
4. a. Extensor digitorum brevis
5. h. Flexor hallucis brevis
6. c. Abductor hallucis
7. j. Adductor hallucis
8. f. Lumbricals pedis
9. i. Flexor digiti minimi pedis
10. l. Dorsal interossei pedis
11. b. Extensor hallucis brevis
12. d. Abductor digiti minimi pedis

Matching Attachments

1. Extensor digitorum brevis
2. Extensor hallucis brevis
3. Abductor hallucis
4. Abductor digiti minimi pedis
5. Flexor digitorum brevis
6. Lumbricals pedis
7. Quadratus plantae
8. Flexor hallucis brevis
9. Flexor digiti minimi pedis
10. Adductor hallucis
11. Plantar interossei
12. Dorsal interossei pedis

The Big Picture – Functional Groups

1. Flexion of the toes
2. Extension of the toes
3. Adduction of the toes
4. Abduction of the toes

Matching Actions

1. g
2. f
3. i
4. j
5. b
6. a, h
7. c
8. d
9. e
10. l
11. m
12. k

The Long and the Short of It – Exercise 1

1. Shortens
2. Shortens
3. Lengthens
4. Lengthens
5. Shortens

The Long and the Short of It – Exercise 2

1. Shortens: abductor hallucis, abductor digiti minimi pedis, dorsal interossei pedis; Lengthens: adductor hallucis, plantar interossei
2. Shortens: adductor hallucis, plantar interossei; Lengthens: abductor hallucis, abductor digiti minimi pedis, dorsal interossei pedis
3. Shortens: extensor hallucis longus, extensor hallucis brevis; Lengthens: flexor hallucis longus, flexor hallucis brevis
4. Shortens: flexor digitorum longus, flexor digitorum brevis, lumbricals pedis, quadratus plantae, flexor digiti minimi pedis; Lengthens: extensor digitorum longus, extensor digitorum brevis, lumbricals pedis
5. Shortens: flexor hallucis longus, flexor hallucis brevis; Lengthens: extensor hallucis longus, extensor hallucis brevis

Movers & Antagonists – Exercise 1

1. Adductor hallucis/Abductor hallucis
2. Flexor digitorum brevis/Extensor digitorum longus
3. Fourth dorsal interosseus pedis/Second plantar interosseus
4. First plantar interosseus/Second dorsal interosseus pedis

Movers & Antagonists – Exercise 2

1. Extensors: contracting; Flexors: relaxed; Type of contraction: concentric
2. Abductors: contracting; Adductors: relaxed; Type of contraction: concentric
3. Adductors: contracting; Abductors: relaxed; Type of contraction: concentric

Muscle Stabilizations

1. a. Plantar interossei
2. c. Dorsal interossei pedis
3. d. Flexor digiti minimi pedis
4. c. Extensor hallucis longus

You've Got Nerve!

1. Deep fibular nerve
2. Deep fibular nerve
3. Medial plantar nerve
4. Lateral plantar nerve
5. Medial plantar nerve
6. Medial plantar nerve, lateral plantar nerve
7. Lateral plantar nerve
8. Medial plantar nerve
9. Lateral plantar nerve
10. Lateral plantar nerve
11. Lateral plantar nerve
12. Lateral plantar nerve

Are You Feeling It? – Palpation

1. Dorsal surfaces of the proximal phalanges of toes two through four
2. Proximal, dorsolateral foot
3. Medial side of the foot, near the plantar surface
4. Lateral side of the distal foot, near the plantar surface
5. Flexor digitorum brevis
6. Metatarsophalangeal joint (MTP)
7. Dorsal surface of foot, between metatarsals

Clinically Speaking

1. Abductor hallucis, abductor digiti minimi pedis, flexor digitorum brevis (plantar layer I)
2. Quadratus plantae
3. Opponens hallucis
4. Opponens digiti minimi pedis
5. Wearing shoes
6. Plantar: 3, 4, and 5; dorsal: 2, 3, and 4

Muscle Mash-Up

1. Transverse and oblique
2. Abductor hallucis, abductor digiti minimi pedis, flexor digitorum brevis
3. Quadratus plantae and lumbricals pedis
4. Flexor hallucis brevis, flexor digiti minimi pedis, adductor hallucis
5. Plantar interossei, dorsal interossei pedis
6. Extensor digitorum brevis, extensor hallucis brevis
7. To differentiate that muscle from the same-name instrinsic muscle of the hand
8. Between bones (metatarsals for intrinsic of the foot)
9. Toes two through four
10. Plantar layer I
11. Lumbricals pedis
12. Plantar layer I
13. Plantar layer III

Crossword Puzzle

Across	Down
8 Quadratus plantae	1 Plantar
9 Pedis	2 Sesamoid
10 Shoes	3 Hallucis
11 Two	4 Handy
12 Lumbrical	5 Tuberosity
	6 Adduct
	7 Metatarsals

Mini Case Studies

1. Plantar layer I, abductor hallucis, abductor digiti minimi pedis, flexor digitorum brevis
2. Yes. All three muscles of the plantar layer I and adductor hallucis specifically help stabilize the arch structure of the foot.
3. Go barefoot more often.

Chapters 9–11 Summary Review - Multiple Choice

1. c. Masseter
2. b. Facial (CN VII)
3. d. Trigeminal (CN V)
4. d. It is often stated to be the most powerful muscle in the human body, proportional to its size
5. b. Piriformis
6. c. Femoral
7. c. Adductor magnus
8. a. Knee joint
9. d. Ischial tuberosity
10. d. Eversion
11. c. Tibial